OTOLARYNGOLOGY RESEARCH ADVANCES

VOICE DISORDERS

EPIDEMIOLOGY, TREATMENT APPROACHES AND LONG-TERM OUTCOMES

Otolaryngology Research Advances

Additional books in this series can be found on Nova's website under the Series tab.

Additional e-books in this series can be found on Nova's website under the e-book tab.

OTOLARYNGOLOGY RESEARCH ADVANCES

VOICE DISORDERS

EPIDEMIOLOGY, TREATMENT APPROACHES AND LONG-TERM OUTCOMES

DERRICK WELCH
EDITOR

NOVA BIOMEDICAL

New York

Additional color graphics may be available in the e-book version of this book.

Library of Congress Cataloging-in-Publication Data

ISBN: 978-1-63484-413-0

Library of Congress Control Number: 2015959370

Published by Nova Science Publishers, Inc. † New York

CONTENTS

PREFACE

This book focuses on the epidemiology, treatment and long-term outcomes of voice disorders. The first chapter proposes evidence based therapy for glottal incompetence, which reflects the dysfunction of the vocal folds on voice and swallowing. Chapter Two presents an overview of the epidemiology, diagnosis, management, extraction techniques, adjuvant medical therapy and prevention of laryngeal papillomatosis in children. Chapter Three presents the latest investigation results related to Speech and Language Pathology intervention in childhood dysphonia, and presents assessment protocols and therapeutic approaches commonly used in voice disorders within the pediatric population. Chapter Four provides a voice analysis of primary school pedagogues in the Czech region of Ostrava.

Chapter 1 – The glottal incompetence is a term that, despite being regarded as general, reflects the dysfunction of the vocal folds on voice and swallowing. An incompetent glottis, as the name suggests, results in an asthenic voice, at first. After the onset of the disorder, patients can develop compensations, even involuntary ones, intending to bring the voice to a normal state. The lack of literature to assist the clinical decision making in these areas, especially concerning glottal incompetence, is palpable. Often, the solution to glottal incompetence depends on a surgery. The costs, impact and consequences of surgery can sometimes be more than Speech Language Therapy intervention. The authors designed a model based on theory and practice that supports therapeutic decisions about cases with glottal incompetence. In this chapter they present and describe a tool to support therapeutic decision-making when facing a case of glottal incompetence. A Conceptual Classification of Glottal Closure Disorders is proposed, which aims to categorize incomplete glottal closure into glottal incompetence and glottal insufficiency. In addition, an original flowchart is presented supported in bibliographic review and an applied/tested therapy program that was implemented in real cases from a Central Hospital ENT Service. In the flowchart, the Speech and Language Pathology intervention is defined by priorities and described throughout the chapter.

Chapter 2 – Dysphonia is common in children. Its main cause is the abuse or misuse of the voice. Congenital, neoplastic, infectious, neurological or iatrogenic causes are less frequent. Recurrent respiratory papillomatosis is the most common benign neoplasm of the larynx in children and the second most frequent cause (after vocal cord nodules) of childhood hoarseness. It is caused by human papilloma viruses, mainly types 6 and 11. It is characterized by its unpredictable course with tendency to recur and spread after removal. Malignant transformation is infrequent but has been reported to occur. A slowly progressive hoarseness is the key symptom of this pathology. With disease progression, signs of obstructive dyspnoea may occur. Since the disease is infrequent, diagnosis is often forgotten and delayed until respiratory problems become apparent. This chapter presents an overview of the epidemiology, diagnosis, management, extraction techniques, adjuvant medical therapy and prevention of laryngeal papillomatosis in children.

Chapter 3 – Dysphonia is present in a growing number of children, resulting in a negative impact on social interaction and academic proficiency. Although some laryngeal lesions or voice disorders can be found more frequently in children, its physiopathology as well as its functional outcomes are not significantly different from those found in adults. Besides the well known anatomic and physiological differences, the great challenge approaching childhood dysphonia lies in their peculiar social and behavioral characteristics. This chapter aims to present the latest investigation results related to Speech and Language Pathology intervention in childhood dysphonia. Voice development is described. Furthermore, the authors present assessment protocols and therapeutic approaches commonly used in voice disorders within the pediatric population. Early identification and awareness improvement among family and school settings play a key role in voice therapy outcomes. Finally, the authors propose a structured intervention protocol and a summary table presenting the most common laryngeal disorders and their characteristics in childhood dysphonia.

Chapter 4 – *Introduction*: A cultivated vocal performance is one of the preconditions of succeeding in many professions. It is mainly used and hence strained by voice professionals for whom it is a work tool. An important group representing voice professionals is composed of pedagogues. The objective of the thesis was a voice analysis of primary school pedagogues in the Czech region of Ostrava.

Methodology: A two-phase study was executed at Ostrava primary schools involving a computer voice analysis performed by means of the lingWAVES computer modular system for voice analysis and therapy. Participation in both phases of the study was based on voluntariness. In the first phase of the study 63 primary schools were approached. 34 primary schools from various city boroughs joined the project between September and November 2012, giving 495 respondents in total. 484 persons underwent an acoustic computer analysis of the voice, which is 98 per cent of respondents. Within the scope of the study's second phase the data collection took place in the second half of June 2013 with 2 primary schools from Poruba joining the project. The lower number in comparison with the first phase is caused by the pedagogues' commitments at the end of the school term, and by part of schools refusing to participate due to specifically abridged school terms. Altogether 19 respondents of the female sex were examined. The final comparison and results of the study included the same pedagogues as in the first and second phase of the study. The data was evaluated using statistical methods.

Results: By means of acoustic assessment of the speaking voice the following was judged – phonation time, intensity range, speaking profile and the vospector DSI (Dysphonia Severity Index). The difference in the results of phonation time between the two phases was insignificant. As regards intensity range and the speaking profile slope, a decrease in the quality of good voices was observed in the second phase of measuring. It is clear from the vospector DSI comparison that there is a difference between the first and second phase of the study in the number of pedagogues in groups 1 (constant dysphonia), 2 (moderate dysphonia), and 3 (slight to medium dysphonia).

Conclusion: The thesis considered the voice quality state by means of focusing on voice professionals, particularly primary school pedagogues. The most significant deterioration in voice quality was recorded in the vospector DSI parameter, where the number of pedagogues in the groups of constant, moderate and medium to slight dysphonia increased. The results of the study confirm both a decline in voice dynamics and voice deterioration at the end of the school term. The project was funded through the grant SMO 0211/2012/KZ: "Epidemiological study of the frequency of voice disorders in pedagogues and a proposal for its prevention" of the University of Ostrava and the Statutory City of Ostrava. The thesis should motivate voice professionals to take preventive measures and thus lower the number of injuries of the vocal apparatus.

In: Voice Disorders
Editor: Derrick Welch
ISBN: 978-1-63484-413-0

Chapter 1

GLOTTAL INCOMPETENCE: PROPOSAL OF AN EVIDENCE BASED THERAPY

Susana Vaz-Freitas*[*], *SLP, MSc, PhD,* *and Pedro Melo Pestana, SLP
Speech Therapy Department of Otolaryngology Service,
Centro Hospitalar do Porto, Porto, Portugal
PMP Terapia, Esposende, Portugal

ABSTRACT

The glottal incompetence is a term that, despite being regarded as general, reflects the dysfunction of the vocal folds on voice and swallowing.

An incompetent glottis, as the name suggests, results in an asthenic voice, at first. After the onset of the disorder, patients can develop compensations, even involuntary ones, intending to bring the voice to a normal state.

The lack of literature to assist the clinical decision making in these areas, especially concerning glottal incompetence, is palpable. Often, the solution to glottal incompetence depends on a surgery. The costs, impact and consequences of surgery can sometimes be more than Speech Language Therapy intervention.

[*] Email: svazfreitas@gmail.com.

The authors designed a model based on theory and practice that supports therapeutic decisions about cases with glottal incompetence. In this chapter they present and describe a tool to support therapeutic decision-making when facing a case of glottal incompetence. A Conceptual Classification of Glottal Closure Disorders is proposed, which aims to categorize incomplete glottal closure into glottal incompetence and glottal insufficiency.

In addition, an original flowchart is presented supported in bibliographic review and an applied/tested therapy program that was implemented in real cases from a Central Hospital ENT Service. In the flowchart, the Speech and Language Pathology intervention is defined by priorities and described throughout the chapter.

Keywords: glottal incompetence, voice therapy, decision making, protocol

INTRODUCTION

The voice is a phenomenon that involves large variations (Le Huche and Allali, 2010) and depends on a complex and interdependent activity of all muscles that allows its production, as well as the integrity of the tissues of the vocal tract (Behlau, 2001).

It is produced through the vocal tract, initiating in the larynx, with the air passage through the vocal folds and the movement of phonoarticulatory structures. To produce speech sounds the vocal folds should be in adduction position (closure). Once the subglottic pressure generated by the respiratory system overcomes the resistance caused by vocal fold adduction, compressed air is released in the supraglottic space, i.e., in the vocal tract, involving the abduction (opening) of the folds.

The glottal incompetence is a term that, although comprehensive, reflects the impact that the dysfunction of the vocal folds have in a voice. An incompetent glottis, as the name suggests, results in hypophonic voice initially.

After the onset of dysphonia compensations may be developed, even involuntarily, which aims to approach the pathological voice to the normal one - which rarely happens fully. (Pinho et al. 2006, Guimarães, 2007).

The lack of literature to assist clinical decisions regarding vocal disorders, especially the glottal incompetence, is large. Often the decision to try to resolve the incompetence results in surgery. The impact, consequences and the ongoing costs, can often be higher than the Speech Therapy intervention.

It is intended, with this chapter, todprovide tools to make the best therapeutic decision when the therapist has a case of glottal incompetence. In addition, we propose an original intervention protocol that has been proved effective.

Conceptual Classification of Glottic Closure Disorders

The glottal closure dysfunction "is a pathological condition characterized by reduced efficient vibration of the vocal fold in a normal aerodynamic support context. It may be due to a decrease of glottal adduction, decreased volume of the vocal fold, altered viscoelasticity of the vocal fold, or a combination of the three" (Ford and Cooper, 2009).

Therefore, normal oscillations of the vocal folds are compromised, and requires larger subglottic pressure and a larger flow of air to be able to start, maintain and enhance the sound production. The usual complaints are vocal fatigue (phonoasthenia), reduced projection and breathy quality (Ford and Cooper, 2009 Pinho et al., 2006).

Glottal closure disorders are common and varied. They can be characterized by the following designations: (Behlau et al., 2005) paralysis and paresis of the vocal folds, atrophy and presbylarynx, loss of soft tissue and scars, or some combination of these conditions. The intervention adopted by the Speech and Language Pathologist varies. The main factors conditioning the goal of therapy are the laryngeal findings, therefore, for authors it makes sense divide the glottal closure disorders in glottal incompetence and glottal insufficiency (see Figure 1). Although in both the function is affected, the intervention will be quite different from one another, starting with the goals.

The glottal incompetence is characterized by a decrease or absence of uni- or bilateral movement of the vocal folds/larynx. In a later and chronic phase you may observe an accentuated decrease or absence of tonus (Bielamowicz et al., 1995, and Hirano and Mori, 2000). Once the change stems from neurological injury or from the disuse, there is no decrease in mass of the vocal folds. In this function changes paralysis or paresis are included, the cricoarytenoid cartilage fixation, the muscle atrophy by disuse and the presbyphonia (Pinho et al., 2006).

Other disturbances may cause glottal incompetence, such as spasmodic dysphonia and Parkinson's disease - in this case, it is not caused by the inability to occlude the glottis but by the inherent involuntary movements.

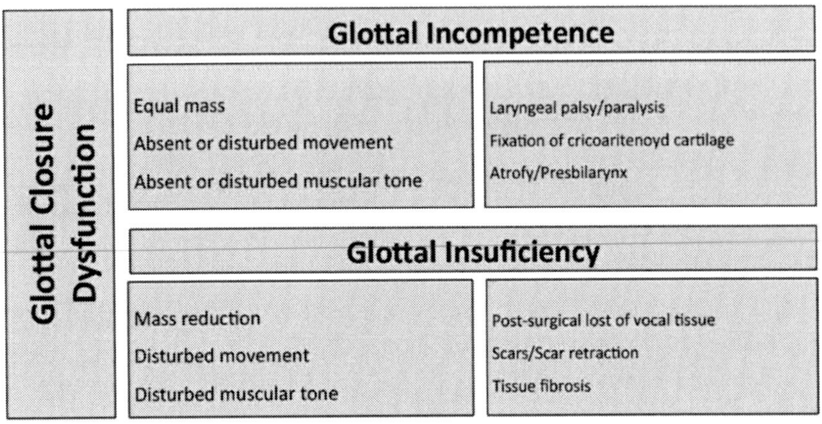

Figure 1. Conceptual Classification of Glottal Closure Disorders.

The presbylarynx, a cause of presbyphonia, despite being a normal process of vocal aging, is characterized by atrophy of the intrinsic muscles of the larynx and loss of tonus and / or edema of the lamina propria, becoming less dense, elastic and fibrotic and prone to atrophy. In addition to causing oval shape glottal gap, during this stage a water deficiency occurs, with the loss of elasticity of the ligaments and cartilage calcification (Ford and Cooper, 2009, Ferreira and Annunciato, 2003).

The concept of glottal insufficiency suggests, immediately, a decrease in mass of the vocal folds. The movement, although always present, may be decreased (narrowed) or slowed. The tonus is altered but never absent. This category includes loss of tissue in post-surgery, scars, retraction scars and tissue fibrosis (Ford and Cooper, 2009).

The authors will focus on a direct therapy protocol regarding the glottal incompetence. A flowchart will be presented to show the various steps taken during the intervention in this laryngeal condition. A standard intervention protocol, which saw its efficiency proven in a group of patients with vocal fold paralysis, is suggested (Pestana, Vaz-Freitas and Almeida, 2012).

Therapeutic Decisions in Glottal Incompetence

The construction of the following flowchart aims to support the therapeutic decisions made when a therapist is faced with a functional diagnosis of glottal incompetence. It will be explained step-by-step based in the Figure 2, shown below.

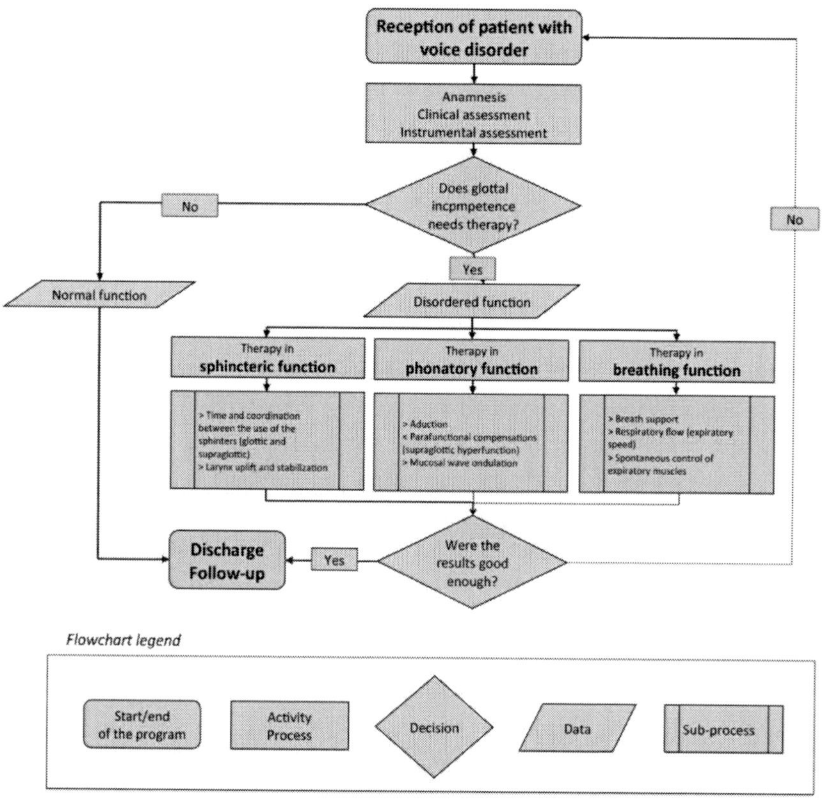

Figure 2. Flowchart of Decision Making Process on Glottal Incompetence.

The process starts with the patient's with voice complaints admission, which seeks therapy or is referred by other clinician (A) (Behlau, 2001; Guimarães, 2007).

The first procedure (B) is the collection of personal data as well as the relevant medical history and lifestyle of the patient (anamnesis). The audio-perceptual and acoustic assessment should be the next step as well as descriptive reports of the exams (e.g., laryngoscopy, etc.) done in this first appointment. It is also at this stage that the Speech and Language Pathologist is responsible for screening other functional disorders, such as dysarthria or other that may affect the intervention and its goals. Contact with other professionals who follow the case should be done if there is any relevant doubt that could affect therapy.

It is then time to identify, evaluate and classify the functional change that the patient has. This flowchart is applicable to all patients who at this stage are identified with glottal incompetence. If this happens we need to verify the necessity for intervention (C). The clinician should never forget to characterize the impact that voice disorder may have in the patient quality of life (Berg et al., 2008, Guimarães, 2007). Another factor that interferes with the prognosis is the time that has elapsed since the establishment of the injury / disorder and / or its evolution (Pinho et al., 2006).

When considering a case where the function is adequate (no significant change) (C.1), if you are not putting the patient at risk or if meeting the patient's expectations, it should be considered to release the patient or do a follow-up (E).

There is a need for intervention whenever at least one glottis dependent function is significantly disturbed or there is a negative impact in the final vocal quality (C.2). In the flowchart, the action is defined by priorities. Thus, the therapist should identify the aspiration or penetration of solid or liquid foods (this last the most frequent), since the safety of the patient comes before any other goals. Thus, in case of dysphagia, the sphincter function should be the one that we first deal with (C2.1). This is supported by doing a FEES (flexible endoscopic evaluation of swallowing) or other instrumental assessment, together with the clinical evaluation. At this point be aware of the possibility of sensitivity alterations (due to the superior laryngeal nerve injury) which is difficult to diagnose – important to use the FEESST (flexible endoscopic evaluation of swallowing - sensory test) - but with significant association to penetration and tracheobronchial aspiration. Generally, the goals of this first phase of the intervention are: to increase the closure length of time and coordination of glottic and supraglottic sphincters, increased elevation and stabilization of the larynx.

At the same time that the professional attends the risk of penetration / aspiration due to the glottal incompetence, he continues with the intervention in phonation (C2.2). At this stage, in line with those of the patients, the overall objectives are: increase glottal adduction, decrease parafunctional compensation during phonation (supraglottic hyperfunction), increase normotensive mucosal wave. Note that there are rare cases with glottal incompetence due to bilateral lesion of the recurrent nerve, where the presented paralysis affects both vocal folds, which are in paramedian position. The therapeutic approach includes advice to vocal rest, to promote atrophy and develop a glottal gap that allows respiratory efficiency. The voice quality is, usually, acceptable.

Glottal incompetence often brings another problem - the inability to resist the passage of expiratory flow during phonation - consistent with the diagnosis of glottal gap that leads to a breathy voice and dyspnoea, in variable degree. There are cases where the phonation is almost non-existent, for example cases of larger glottal gaps and /or in paralysis widely separated from the median position. So, in these patients the intervention goals regarding respiratory function should be: increase respiratory support for speech, increase expiratory flow (exhalation rate) and increase of the voluntary control of the expiratory muscles.

After therapy conclusion the clinician should, together with the patient/family, verify if the results where good (D). This decision must be made based on a reassessment. If the intervention has been successful, the patient should be discharged from therapy or do a follow-up within a time set, to control the larynx characteristics as well as the functional consequences in voice, breathing and swallowing. If the results are unsatisfactory, the therapist should rethink therapy and the evolution of the patient. Therapy should continue until one or more of the following criteria is achieved: 1) normal voice/similar to premorbid; 2) sufficient voice, though disordered, for social and professional demanding; 3) recovery of complaints on sphincter and respiratory functions.

Evidence Based Therapy Protocol

The therapy protocol results from the experience of a decade working in a central hospital in the north of Portugal, in which a hundred cases with unilateral or bilateral vocal fold paralysis were followed.

The assessment is initially made in a phoniatric appointment by a multidisciplinary team: Otolaryngologyst and the Speech and Language Pathologist. Clinical voice assessment includes the collection of information through: clinical interview, assessment of laryngeal physiology, audio-perceptual evaluation, muscle-skeletal and aerodynamic functional examination, acoustical analysis and self-assessment of the impact of voice in quality of life (Sousa et al., 2011, Vaz- Freitas, 2009).

In a study made by Pestana, Vaz-Freitas and Almeida (2012) a group of 38 individuals who did Speech Therapy was analysed, using assessment data from the beginning and the end of treatment. Before therapy, on average, fundamental frequency was 206.74 Hz (see Table I). In general there was a tendency to increase its value in the post-therapy assessment. However, the difference is not significant. Based on the standard deviation it can be stated that the variability of data, on both occasions, was considerable. On the other hand, differences in results of the other acoustic parameters (jitter, shimmer, NNE) was statistically significant ($p < 0.05$).

The jitter (local) was outside the normal average, pre-therapy. By analysing mean results obtained post-therapy it can be concluded that they were closer to normal (i.e., slightly above 0), by accepting that any voice is somewhat unstable, so jitter may vary between 0.5 and 1.0%. The differences between the results in the two times are, as mentioned above, statistically significant (see Table I).

Similar results, but less pronounced, were found for shimmer (local). There was a decrease post- therapy and the values were closer to normal (see Table I). The investigations on this topic suggests that this measurement is inversely proportional to the average intensity, i.e., the bigger this is, the lower the shimmer value, and vice versa. This measure provides an indirect perception of noise on voice signal. Thus, in voice disorders shimmer appears more changed in low frequencies and low intensity – which is common in vocal fold paralysis.

The shimmer measures may be presented in different forms (Pinho et al., 2006; Pouchoulin, 2008) one of which is in percentage (directional disturbance factor). The commonly used threshold value is 3.0% (Yu et al., 2001), or 5.0% (0.44 dB) (Lindsey, 1997 in Pinho et al., 2006). It represents the amplitude variation of consecutive periods using the average value of the amplitude contained in the segment being analysed, i.e., measures the number of times that the amplitude difference between consecutive cycles changes direction. From here we can conclude that there was a decrease in the production of noise during emission – which also suggests, in concordance with Behlau (2001), that there was a decrease in breathiness.

The Normalized Noise Energy (NNE) achieved results that are statistically significant different. The pre-treatment results were quite inadequate, revealing, as mentioned by Behlau (2001) "aperiodic phonation". The therapy resulted in values closer to normal, i.e., above -10dB (see Table I).

Table 1. Results of acoustic analysis pre- and post-therapy
(Pestana, Vaz-Freitas and Almeida, 2012)

Acoustic Measure	Pre-Therapy	Post-Therapy
F_0 (Hz)	206.74±59.86	212.72±59.80
Jitter (%)	1.023±0.98	0.44±0.70**
Shimmer (%)	6.73±5.91	3.11±3.11**
NNE (dB)	-5.64±4.63	-9.55±6.17**

Data are presented using mean ± standard deviation; ** $p < 0.05$ comparing pre- and post-therapy – Wilcoxon Test; F_0 = mean fundamental frequency; NNE = normalized noise energy.

The timings for therapy and the adopted methods and techniques were effective when the following conditions were met (Benninger et al., 1994; Pinho et al., 2006):

1. Timing between the onset of complaints and begin therapy - most accompanied cases were evaluated in the first week after installation of symptoms of swallowing / voice / breathing. All patients were scheduled to repeat laryngeal observation and start therapy within a month.
2. Unilateral or bilateral glottic impairment - traditionally the most severe cases were those with a bilateral disorder, highlighting that position of the paralysis implies an adjustment of therapy goals.
3. The degree of the voice and swallowing disorder - voice quality in unilateral paralysis is easily recognizable. Most patients report symptoms: difficulty in vocal projection, breathiness, voice instability and asthenia, frequent choking with liquids and/or their own saliva.
4. Availability of patient to come to appointments and ability to understand the given guidelines - the protocol is based on the need for short but frequent repetition of a set of motor acts, so its effectiveness is based on isotonic and isometric muscle work. At the beginning of therapy – since it is new to the patient patient - if possible, we recommend bi-weekly appointments. Each and every therapy exercise should be based on demonstration, using strategies such as modelling, so the patient can repeat accordingly in their own context. Speech and Language Pathologist guidelines and oral explanations benefit of a written and graphic support.

This protocol is based on the use of motor tasks with immediate impact in glottal adduction, thus improving phonation and glottal sphincter ability (Behlau, 2005; Behlau, 2010; Guimarães, 2007; Pinho et al., 2006). It is up to the clinician to adjust the intensity and/or frequency of therapy according with the needs and difficulties of the patient. Examples are: a patient who has difficulty swallowing liquids because of a unilateral paralysis of the larynx easily benefits from postural manoeuvre of head rotation; a patient with comorbidities – cervical joints and bone limitations – may not carry some of the postural techniques.

The therapy plan is organized into eight weeks, with initial bi-weekly visits, making an average of 13.29 hours of direct therapy (Pestana, Vaz-Freitas and Almeida, 2012), two of them to assess, in the beginning and end of treatment (Pinho et al., 2006). Exercises are performed in-office and the patient gets a prescription workout plan to repeat daily, every two hours, for ten minutes. The materials needed are: the prescription, a chair, a mirror.

1st Week: in the first week the voice therapy exercises use the reflex mechanism of glottal adduction with no sound associated to head and lower limbs movements. The patient should be seated and comply with a moment of inspiratory apnoea, within five seconds, during which assuming different positions of the head, in different directions, or movements of the lower limbs, individually or at the same time. In addition to the visual support with photos, you also need to readjust vocabulary in your descriptions of the exercises the patient needs to follow.

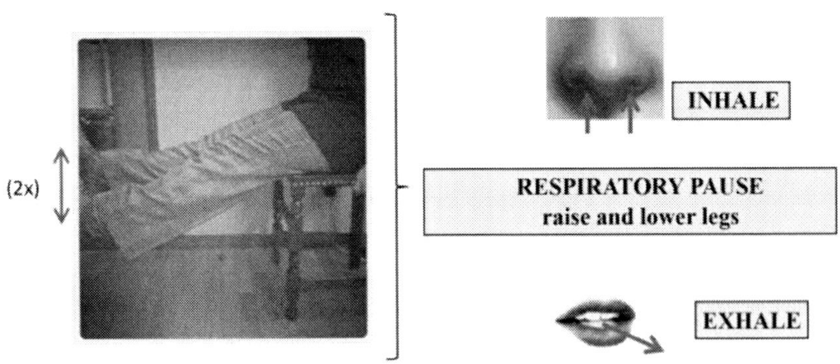

Figure 3. Example of Therapy Exercise from Week 1.

2nd Week: in the second week the exercises are based on the movement of the head with audible sounds. Therefore, combining the variation of the head position in the various plans (after maintenance within 5 seconds inspiratory apnoea) with the production of specific voiced sounds, during expiration, in maximum phonation time. You can also use a fixed head posture, namely the rotation for the injured side or the inclination to the other as phonation facilitators. There may also be used pairs or combinations of sounds as an alternative to isolated. When there are difficulties in maintaining voicing, it can be easier to produce vowels, namely diphthongs such as: [ai], [au], [ua], [ui], [iu], [ia].

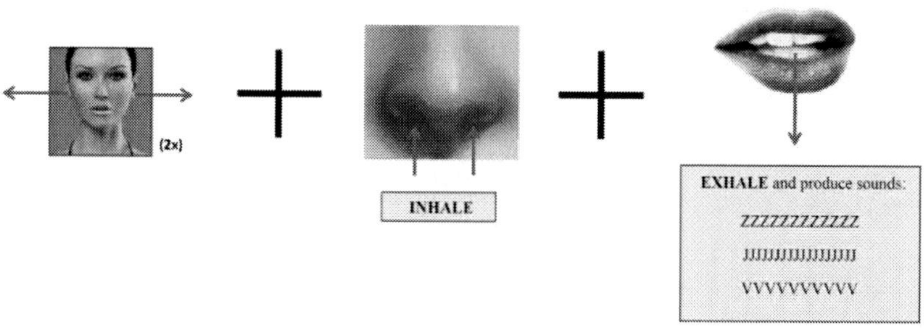

Figure 4. Example of Therapy Exercise from Week 2.

3rd Week: in third week emphasis is placed on the vocal strength by performing pushing and pulling exercises/effort. Fixed positions of the upper limbs during inspiratory apnoea are stimulated, and then the production of monosyllables with plosives - unvoiced and voiced - associated with open vowels [a], [E], [O], in loud voice.

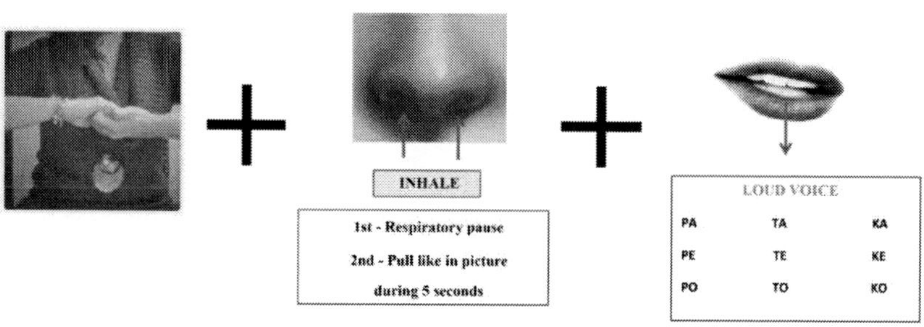

Figure 5. Example of Therapy Exercise from Week 3.

4th Week: the only difference from the above is the syllabic reduplication. Patients are able to voice longer, therefore they may produce dissyllabic and multisyllabic words with voice projection. Note that the movement of pushing/pulling effort can now be standing, sitting or even lying down. Lists of words for training can be built with the patient. At this stage the patient can keep training the previous exercises alternating them along in the different times of daily practice.

5th Week: in this week we start favouring tasks closer to spontaneous speech, or reading of texts. In this prevail sounds included in the previous weeks of therapy, including sibilants (for sustaining) and plosives, unvoiced and voiced (for vocal projection). Besides reading with the use of these techniques, we also may use sounds with frequency variation and inspiratory phonation. You can also use a midline fixed head posture, the rotation of the head to the injured side or tilted to the normal side.

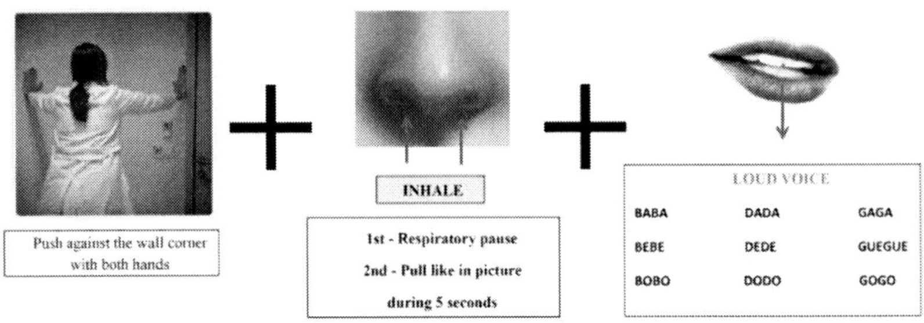

Figure 6. Example of Therapy Exercise from Week 4.

Sound V

Vincent vowed vengeance very vehemently.

Figure 7. Example of Therapy Exercise from Week 5 (for sound sustaining).

Sound P

Peter poked a poker at the piper, so the piper poked pepper at Peter.

Figure 8. Example of Therapy Exercise from Week 5 (for sound projection).

6st Week: refers to a set of exercises to increase vocal resistance to sound production, using semi-occluded vocal tract techniques. Some of the possibilities are finger kazoo (Behlau, 2005) or the production of sound to a straw (Resonance Tube Technique) (Laukkanen et al., 2008; Sampaio et al., 2008). It is possible to scale the output resistance of the blow/sound (e.g., by varying the number of fingers in the finger kazoo or decreasing the lumen of the straws). Sounds [u] and [v] can be produced isolated in maximum phonation time, with pitch variation (glissando) or associated with a musical rhythm (melody). In this week vibration sounds associated with different head positions or movement, in different planes, can be used. There is a higher effectiveness of tongue base vibration, although some cases refer laryngeal irritability and altered vocal quality immediately after the exercise, with short-term and easily recovered hoarseness.

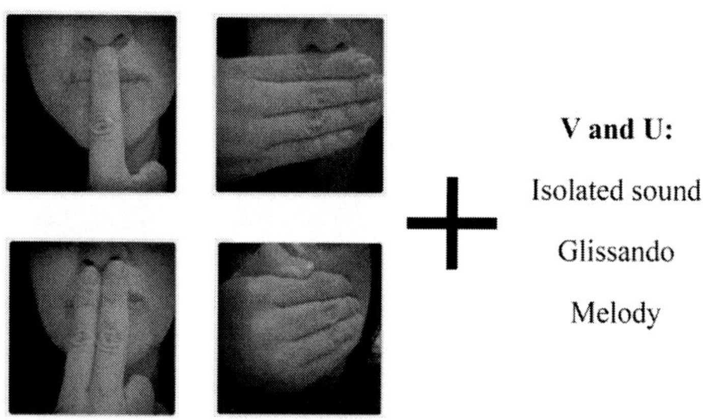

Figure 9. Example of Therapy Exercise from Week 6.

7th Week: the patient should already be able to have an audible voice, sustained and very similar to previous normal voice quality. However, there are common complaints like: difficulty in extreme frequencies (usually higher notes) and sudden and unpredictable pitch variations. Thus the focus is reading with speech techniques such as mesa di voce, pitch and loudness variations and chanted voice (Pinho and Pontes, 2008). There is also the need to prioritize the difficulty of the exercises, starting with the variation between sentences to the changes applied between each word.

LOUD VOICE - Everyone suspects himself of at least one of the cardinal virtues

WEAK VOICE . Hand to hand is how it will be, a life and death fight against the fiend

Figure 10. Example of Therapy Exercise from Week 7.

8th Week: the eighth week concerns the maintenance of all acquisitions made so far. The only complexity lies in sound juncture used in selected texts - the tongue twisters are frequently used. In these apply the different techniques used in previous weeks. Namely, sustaining facilitator sounds (sibilants, vibrant, nasal, etc), change in pitch and loudness, inspiratory phonation, chanted voice, among others.

CONCLUSION

The effective role of therapy regarding voice disorders is commonly accepted. However there aren`t so many studies that prove it.

The methods and techniques adopted have proved to be effective (Pestana, Vaz-Freitas and Almeida, 2012), corroborating evidence of its application in this pathology. It can be said that through therapy other procedures such as surgeries were not necessary to compensate the voice disorder.

Difference between objective measures - before and after therapy - is statistically significant, so this chapter reinforces that fulfilling this evidence based therapy protocol results in positive, clinical and functional, outcomes.

ACKNOWLEDGMENTS

The authors acknowledge the collaboration of patients who contributed to the data that were discussed in this chapter. A mention also to colleague Rita Rosas that provided images of the different techniques used in each week of the therapy plan. We are indebted to Rita Alegria and Fernando Governo for the productive discussion and valuable comments on the manuscript.

REFERENCES

Bach, K. K., Belafsky, P. C., Wasylik, K., Postma, G. N. & Koufman, J. A. 2005. Validity and reliability of the glottal function index. *Arch Otolaryngol Head Neck Surg*, 131, 961-4.

Behlau, M. 2001. A Voz: o Livro do Especialista, São Paulo.

Behlau, M. 2005. A Voz: o Livro do Especialista, São Paulo.

Behlau, M. 2010. Técnicas Vocais. In: Fernandes, F., Mendes, B. & Navas, A. (eds.) Tratado de Fonoaudiologia. São Paulo: Roca.

Benninger, M. S., Crumley, R. L., Ford, C. N., Gould, W. J., Hanson, D. G., Ossoff, R. H. & Sataloff, R. T. 1994. Evaluation and treatment of the unilateral paralyzed vocal fold. *Otolaryngol Head Neck Surg*, 111, 497-508.

Berg, E., Hapner, E., Klein, A. & Johnsiii, M. 2008. Voice Therapy Improves Quality of Life in Age-Related Dysphonia: A Case-Control Study. *Journal of Voice*, 22, 70-74.

Bielamowicz, S., Berke, G. S. & Gerratt, B. R. 1995. A comparison of type I thyroplasty and arytenoid adduction. *J Voice*, 9, 466-72.

Ferreira, L. M. & Annunciato, N. F. 2003. Envelhecimento Vocal e Neuroplasticidade. In: Pinho, S. (ed.) Fundamentos em Fonoaudiologia - Tratando os Distúrbios da Voz. 2ª ed. Rio de Janeiro: Guanabara Koogan.

Ford, C. N. & Cooper, K. A. 2009. Management of Vocal Fold Incompetence with Vocal Fold Injectable Fillers. In: Blitzer, A., Brin, M. F. & Ramig, L. O. (eds.) Neurologic Disorders of the Larynx. New York: Thieme.

Guimarães, I. 2007. A Ciência e Arte da Voz Humana, Alcoitão, ESSA.

Hirano & Mori 2000. Vocal Fold Paralysis. In: Kent, R. & Ball, M. (eds.) Voice Quality Measurement. Singular Pub. Group.

Laukkanen, A. M., Titze, I. R., Hoffman, H. & Finnegan, E. 2008. Effects of a semioccluded vocal tract on laryngeal muscle activity and glottal adduction in a single female subject. *Folia Phoniatr Logop*, 60, 298-311.

Le Huche, F. & Allali, A. 2010. La voix: Anatomie et physiologie des organes de la voix et de la parole, Paris, Elsevier Masson.

Pestana, P., Vaz-Freitas, S. & Sousa, C. 2012. A Eficácia da Intervenção em Terapia da Fala na Paralisia da Corda Vocal: Avaliação Objectiva. Revista da Sociedade Portuguesa de Otorrinolaringologia, 50(3): 215-220.

Pinho, S. & Pontes, P. 2008. Músculos Intrínsecos Da Laringe E Dinâmica Vocal, Rio de Janeiro, Revinter.

Pinho, S., Tsuji, D. & Bohadana, S. 2006. Fundamentos em Laringologia e Voz, São Paulo, Revinter.

Pouchoulin, G. 2008. Approche Statistique pour L`Analyse Objective et la Caractérisation de la Voix Dysphonique. Université d`Avignon et des Pays de Vaucluse.

Sampaio, M., Oliveira, G. & Behlau, M. 2008. Investigação de efeitos imediatos de dois exercícios de trato vocal semi-ocluído. Pró-Fono Revista de Atualização Científica, 20.

Sousa, R., Vaz-Freitas, S. & Ferreira, A. 2011. A avaliação acústica da voz nas práticas profissionais dos terapeutas da fala portugueses. Revista da Sociedade Portuguesa de Otorrinolaringologia, 49.

Vaz-Freitas, S. 2009. A Avaliação das Alterações Vocais: Registo e Análise Audio-perceptual e Acústica da Voz. In: Peixoto, V. & Rocha, J. (eds.) Metodologias de Intervenção em Terapia da Fala. Porto: Edições Universidade Fernando Pessoa.

Yu, P., Ouaknine, M., Revis, J. & Giovanni, A. 2001. Objective voice analysis for dysphonic patients: a multiparametric protocol including acoustic and aerodynamic measurements. *J Voice*, 15, 529-42.

In: Voice Disorders
Editor: Derrick Welch

ISBN: 978-1-63484-413-0

Chapter 2

RECURRENT RESPIRATORY PAPILLOMATOSIS IN CHILDREN

***Giselle Cuestas*[1,*], *Dr*,**
***Juan Agustín Rodríguez D'Aquila*[2], *Dr*,**
***Máximo Rodríguez D'Aquila*[3], *Dr*,**
and Hugo Rodríguez*[4], *Dr

[1]Otolaryngologist, Otolaryngology Department,
Hospital Italiano de Buenos Aires, Buenos Aires, Argentina;
[2]Otolaryngologist, Centro OIR, Buenos Aires, Argentina
[3]Otolaryngologist, Otolaryngology Department,
Fundación Arauz, Buenos Aires, Argentina
[4]Pediatric Otolaryngologist, Chief of Respiratory Endoscopic Department,
Hospital de Pediatría Prof. Dr. Juan P Garrahan, Buenos Aires, Argentina

ABSTRACT

Dysphonia is common in children. Its main cause is the abuse or misuse of the voice. Congenital, neoplastic, infectious, neurological or iatrogenic causes are less frequent.

Recurrent respiratory papillomatosis is the most common benign neoplasm of the larynx in children and the second most frequent cause (after vocal cord nodules) of childhood hoarseness. It is caused by human

* Corresponding Author E mail: giselle_cuestas@yahoo.com.ar.

papilloma viruses, mainly types 6 and 11. It is characterized by its unpredictable course with tendency to recur and spread after removal. Malignant transformation is infrequent but has been reported to occur.

A slowly progressive hoarseness is the key symptom of this pathology. With disease progression, signs of obstructive dyspnoea may occur. Since the disease is infrequent, diagnosis is often forgotten and delayed until respiratory problems become apparent.

This chapter presents an overview of the epidemiology, diagnosis, management, extraction techniques, adjuvant medical therapy and prevention of laryngeal papillomatosis in children.

Keywords: dysphonia, laryngeal papillomatosis, management

INTRODUCTION

Recurrent respiratory papillomatosis (RRP) is a disease of viral origin that affects both children and adults with different levels of aggressiveness and severity.

It is a rare disease of the aerodigestive tract caused by human papilloma virus (HPV), mainly types 6 and 11 [1, 2]. It is characterized by the proliferation of exophytic epithelial lesions, mainly of the larynx [3].

It is the most common benign laryngeal tumor in children and the second most common cause of dysphonia in children after vocal cord nodules [1]. The prevalence of this disease has been estimated to be 1.45 to 2.93 per 100,000 children [4], being higher in low socioeoconomic status populations.

This disease has an unpredictable clinical course, tends to recur and to spread outside the larynx. It may have significant morbidity, and may cause a potentially lethal obstruction or develop into malign neoplasms, mainly due to HPV types 11 and 16 [1].

HPV is vertically transmitted from mother to child through the birth canal (latent genital infection or condylomata acuminata). The presence of genital condylomata in women during labor increases more than 200 times the risk of passing the infection to their newborns [5]. Transmission may also be transplacental (1%), attesting to possible blood transmission through the umbilical cord. Young primiparous mothers, vaginal delivery and being first-born children (75% of affected children) are risk factors for RRP [1]. Prolonged deliveries and the premature rupture of membranes, even two hours before delivery, are also associated with an increased risk of transmission.

DIAGNOSIS

Although infection occurs at birth or before, most patients do not show symptoms immediately.

The diagnosis of papillomatosis is generally delayed due to the subtle onset of symptoms and the lack of clinical suspicion in children, especially in infants. Papillomatosis is commonly diagnosed in children aged 2 to 5 years, generally one year after the onset of symptoms, when dysphonia is marked or when there is stridor and respiratory obstruction [5].

- Signs and symptoms

In 75% of children, symptoms start to develop before age 5 [1]. Since the most common initial site of the disease is the vocal cords, a weak cry or dysphonia are the most important and revealing symptoms. Dysphonia is persistent and progressive, with no periods of normal voice.

As the papillomas increase in size, they start to obstruct the airway, causing progressive respiratory distress and low-pitched inspiratory stridor, which becomes biphasic as the disease progresses.

Other symptoms are: chronic coughing, recurrent respiratory infections, dysphagia and growth retardation [6, 7].

- Endoscopy

Flexible laryngoscopy under local anesthesia allows to visualize the typical well vascularized flat or vegetative lesions, white pinkish in color and looking like warty "grape clusters or strawberries" (Figure 1). It is important to perform an endoscopic assessment under general anesthesia to determine lesion extension (lower airway and esophagus involvement) (Figure 2). The stroboscopic evaluation reveals the typical incomplete and irregular glottal closure, and reduced vibratory amplitude and mucosal wave.

- Anatomic pathology

The certain diagnosis of papillomatosis is provided by a biopsy to identify the histopathological features of the lesion and eventually HPV typification.

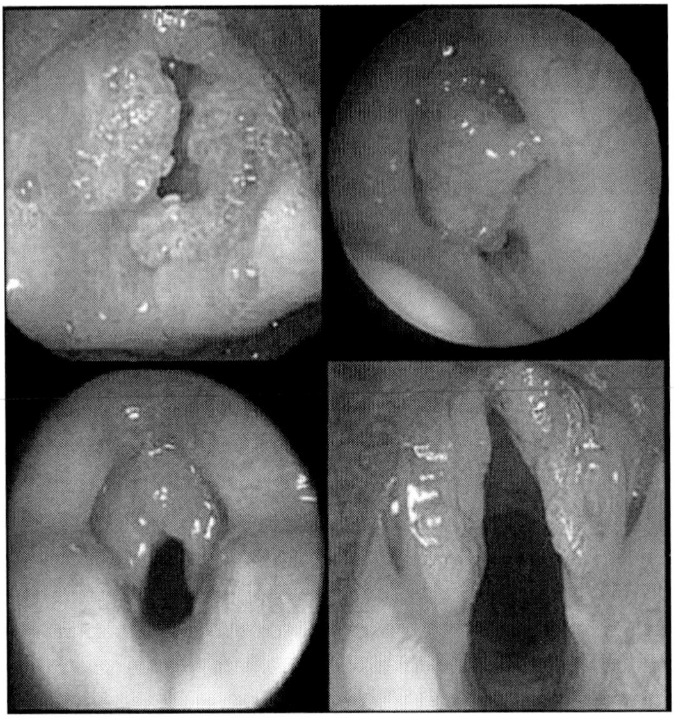

Figure 1. Endoscopic images of laryngeal papillomas.

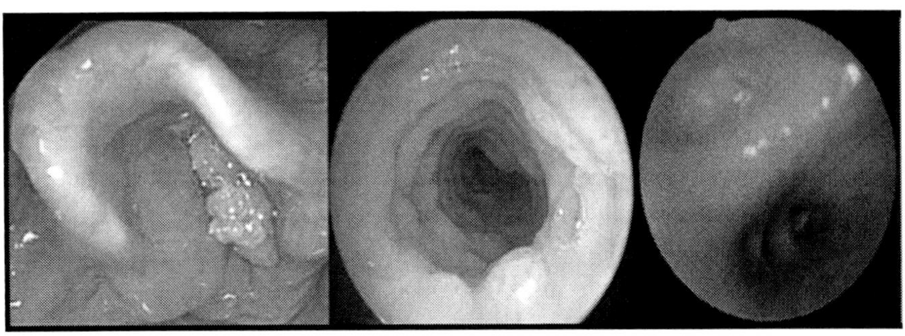

Figure 2. Laryngeal papillomatosis with extralaryngeal dissemination (trachea and bronchi).

Histopathology

HPV mainly causes lesions at transitional epithelium levels (squamous to ciliary epithelia), such as the nasal vestibule, the junction of the oronasopharyngeal mucosa, the supraglottis, the vocal folds and areas of squamous metaplasia such as the tracheal stoma. Papillomas consist of finger-like projections with a central fibrovascular core and a stratified pavement epithelium. The epithelium evidences a delayed maturation that causes thickening of the basal layer with presence of nucleated cells in the superficial layers. The koilocyte is the classical manifestation of cell infection by HPV. It is a squamous epithelial cell, which is often superficial and intermediate, showing typical changes both in its nucleus and cytoplasm. Its shape may be rounded or oval, is characterized by an eccentric cell nucleus. A great cavity or halo, oval in shape or slightly scalloped with well-defined margins, is observed within the cytoplasm (paranuclear halo).

Typification

The viral serotype could be associated with the severity and clinical course of the disease [8, 9]. Determining the viral serology by PCR (polymerase chain reaction) will enable to know the course of the disease according to the serotype and could be useful to identify those patients that due to their viral serology could be at greater risk for recurrence, extralaryngeal spread and malignization. Almost 100 different HPV serotypes have been identified [10]. Studies on the viral identification of RRP, have most frequently detected serotypes 6 and 11 and have observed that the presence of HPV type 11 in the papillomas is associated with an earlier proliferation of larger warts, causing a more obstructive disease than that caused by serotype 6, as well as with higher recurrence rates, greater risk of bronchopulmonary spread and more frequent surgical treatments and adjuvant medication requirement [8-12]. Serotypes 16 and 18 were less frequently isolated but have greater risk of developing cancer [2, 8].

- **Imaging Studies**

A computed tomography scan of the chest should be ordered to assess pulmonary involvement (3%), mainly when tracheal (8%) and/or bronchial (3%) spread of the papillomas is observed (Figure 3). Peripheral nodular lesions can be observed at lung parenchymal level, showing central cavitation or hydroaereal levels, later leading to necrosis, which imply recurrent pneumonias, bronchiectasis and pulmonary function loss, portending an ominous prognosis [1, 5].

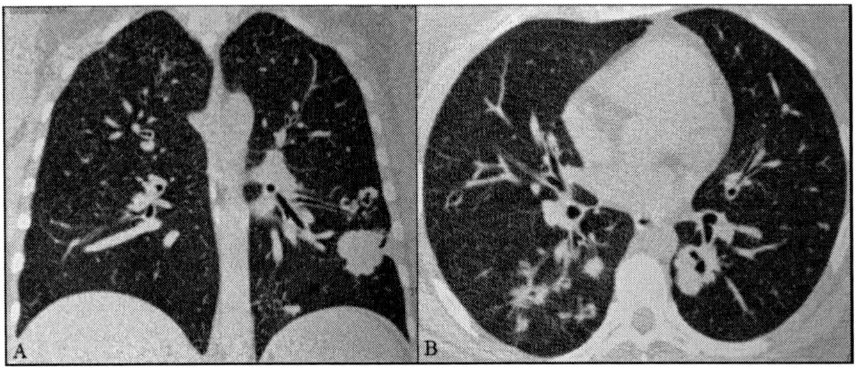

Figure 3. Computed tomography scan of a patient suffering from bronchopulmonary papillomatosis. A. Coronal view. B. Axial view.

Differential Diagnosis

Although most dysphonias in children are due to misuse of the voice, it is important to assess the airway to rule out a tumor growth (benign or malignant), vocal cord paralysis and congenital abnormalities that can be treated with surgery, such as cysts and membranes, among other causes.

Clinical differences between laryngeal papillomatosis and vocal cord nodules:

Children diagnosed with vocal cord nodules have different vocal behavior habits; their voice worsens when they whisper and improves when they shout. Children suffering from papillomatosis exhibit dysphonia that may progress to aphonia over time, showing no voice improvement and concomitant respiratory involvement [1, 6].

Treatment

RRP is a very difficult disease to treat, which despite its low prevalence can have a significant impact on the patients' quality of life as well as on their families. At present no specific treatment has demonstrated to have a curative effect. All currently available treatments, both medical and surgical, are only palliative and aim to secure a safe airway, improve the voice quality, prevent the spread of the disease and increase the time interval between surgeries [3, 6, 13].

• Surgical Treatment

Laryngeal microsurgery can be performed using microscopic or endoscopic surgery equipment, a microdebrider, a CO_2 laser, a KTP laser, micro pincers or forceps.

A tracheostomy should be avoided because it increases the risk of distal tracheal spread extending to the bronchi; however in severe cases it may be necessary [14].

Some common complications of papillomatosis surgery are anterior and posterior commissure synechiae, which cause additional hoarseness and dyspnea, respectively (Figure 4). These scarring processes are frequent in those patients undergoing multiple surgeries, and is the result of the attempt of removing all the lesions present, thus damaging the normal mucosa.

Some small lesions in the anterior and posterior commissures should not be removed (we should bear in mind that papillomatosis is a viral disease and that the virus remains in the mucosal cells) since the treatment and resolution of synechiae is difficult and complicated and requires surgery of an HPV-infected tissue.

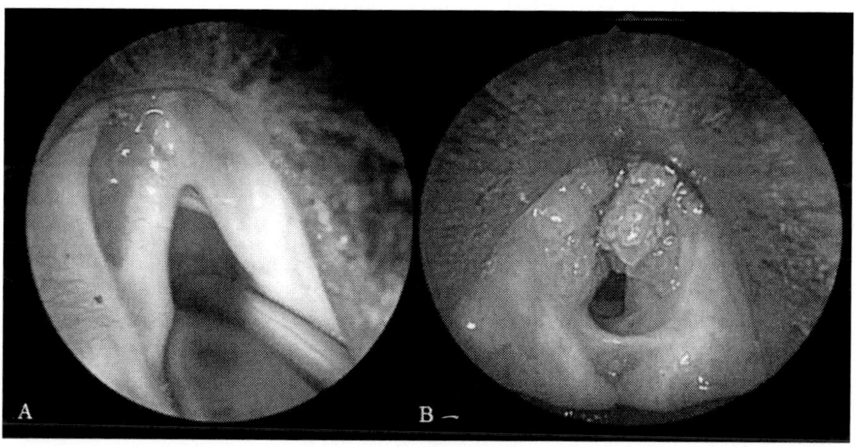

Figure 4. Post-surgical complications of laryngeal papillomatosis. A. Anterior commissure synechia. B. Posterior commissure synechia.

• Adjuvant Medical Treatment

Although RRP is histologically benign, it is potentially lethal and continues to be a frustrating disease to treat due to its high incidence of recurrence [11]. RRP may be a very aggressive disease requiring frequent surgical procedures under general anesthesia for securing a patent airway and for tumor debulking. Adjuvant therapies gained ground in medical practice in an attempt to minimize recurrence and possible complications, to prevent the spread of the disease, to increase the time interval between surgical procedures and to reduce or avoid the need for further surgeries under general anesthesia and possible risks of synechiae and scars, as well as to improve the voice and quality of life.

These adjuvant therapies are used approximately in 25% of affected children [1]. *Adjuvant therapies are indicated in* the following cases [1, 15]:

- More than 4 surgical procedures in a year.
- Children under 2 years of age.
- Need for a tracheostomy.
- Distal spread.
- Fast growth involving respiratory obstruction.
- Anterior or posterior commisure papillomas.

There is controversy regarding the efficacy and side effects of the different adjuvant agents.

Cidofovir (antiviral, nucleotide analog of cytosine) is the most commonly used adjuvant agent [15]. Four intralesional injections of 5 mg/ml, 2 to 4 ml are administered, with a two week interval [16]. Response varies according to viral phenotype, 50% of the strains are susceptible and resolve at the mentioned dose, 30% are intermediate and respond at a dose of 10 mg/ml and finally, 20% are resistant, not responding at any dose [6]. This treatment may not be effective for all children and its use has been associated with several side effects including carcinogenic effects in animal studies; and malignant transformation have been reported in patients suffering from RRP that had received intralesional Cidofovir [17].

When there is no successful response to Cidofovir, a safe and effective option is the use of *Bevacizumab* [18-20]. Vascularization could be a determinant factor influencing the rapid recurrence rate of papillomas. Bevacizumab is a monoclonal antibody targeting the vascular endothelial growth factor. Therefore, it would work as an angiogenesis inhibitor, thus hampering or stopping the growth of papillomas and associated complications [17, 21]. Three to four 2.5 to 5 mg/ml consecutive injections of Bevacizumab are administered approximately every 2 to 3 weeks [22].

Another option is *Alpha-2A Interferon*, which is subcutaneously injected daily to a dose of 5 million U/m2 of body surface area for 28 days, then 3 times weekly for 6 months. The response rate ranges from 30 to 60%. The following side effects have been reported: hepatic dysfunction, neutropenia, anorexia and headaches [1].

Other antiviral drugs prescribed are Ribavirin and Acyclovir. Other described treatments are Indole-3-Carbinol at 100-200 mg/day (dietary supplement present in vegetables such as broccoli, cauliflower and cabbage) and retinoids (1-2 mg/k/day for 6 months).

It is important to monitor all these drugs due to their toxicity and side-effects.

The *treatment for gastroesophageal reflux* disease in patients with laryngeal papillomas may reduce soft tissue complications (synechiae).

Tracheobronchial and pulmonary parenchymal lesions not accesible to local therapies are a great therapeutical challenge. Although RRP mainly affects the larynx, *distal airway spread* may occur.

When RRP affects the pulmonary parenchyma, there are no effective therapeutic strategies, often having a fatal outcome. The systemic administration of Cidofovir is not recommended due to its nephrotoxicity [1]. There were some cases in which the systemic adjuvant therapy using Bevacizumab was associated with intrapulmonary lesion remission and improvement of the symptoms as well as with a decrease in the need for subsequent surgical interventions and lack of severe adverse effects [23, 24].

Evolution

The natural course of the disease is unpredictable. After its onset, some children may experience spontaneous resolution of the papillomas or the disease may remain stable, only requiring sporadic surgical resections. On the other hand, there are rare cases with an aggressive clinical course of fast lesion growth that require frequent surgical interventions to unobstruct the airway (after several days or weeks) and aggressive adjuvant medical treatment, or there may be tracheobronchial and pulmonary involvement or even a malignant transformation of the lesions [10].

The crisis and remission progression pattern is the most frequent. There have been less frequent reports of extralaryngeal spread to the trachea, bronchi, lungs, esophagus and oral cavity (30%); and in rare long-term cases (more than 15 years), of malignant transformation of RRP to squamous cell carcinoma (1%) [1, 5] (Figure 5).

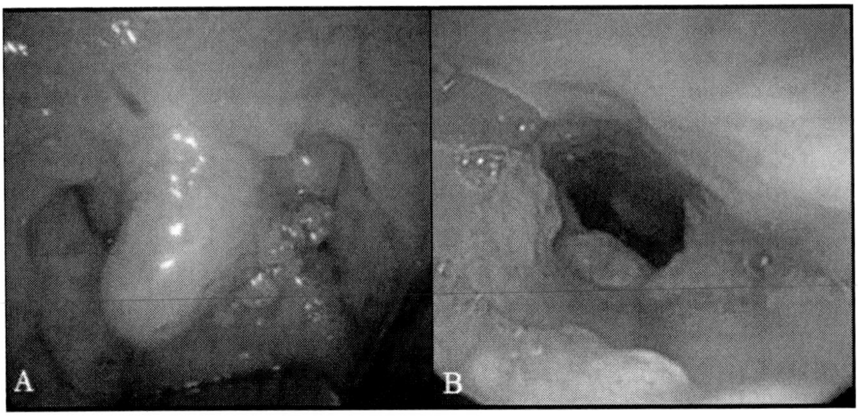

Figure 5. A. Papillomas of the uvula. B. Esophageal papillomatosis.

Papillomatosis and Voice

Benign tumors of the larynx may cause dysphonia due to the direct involvement of the vocal cords or of adjacent structures that interfere with the vocal vibratory function [25].

In a child suffering from RRP, the voice may be affected either by the papillomas or by the administered treatment. The papillomas may cause dysphonia if they compromise the vibratory margin or if the mass effect affects the vibration, hampering the complete glottal closure [25].

When the surgical treatment of laryngeal papillomatosis is performed, its main objective is to secure adequate ventilation to avoid a tracheostomy. However, it should be borne in mind that the preservation of all anatomical structures is vital to optimize the future quality of the voice.

The long-term goal of the surgical treatment of RRP is the preservation of the normal function of the larynx. The papillomas should be carefully removed to preserve the laryngeal function. In many cases, the natural history of the papillomas is the complete resolution of the disease. Surgical intervention therefore must not result in long term complications for either the voice or the airway.

The main reason for performing a surgical procedure is the preservation of a patent and safe airway. The complete resection of all visible papillomas during each surgical procedure is a quite unrealistic and an unnecesary goal, which may lead to permanent damage of the larynx, causing dysphonia or laryngeal stenosis [26]. It is estimated that there is 35% delayed complication rate in the treatment of laryngeal papilloma. The majority of complications are web. Scarring of the true vocal cord, the formation of interarytenoid bands that limit normal abduction of the true vocal cord and fixation of the false vocal cord to the true vocal cord may also occur as a result of the reckless use of any of the surgical procedures available [26].

During the surgical resection of the papillomas, special care should be exercised to preserve the vocal ligament and the mucosa in the anterior and posterior commissures of the larynx so as to avoid synechiae of the vocal cords. When the disease is diffuse and affects anterior and posterior commissures of the larynx, all papillomas should be resected except those located in the commissures. Cidofovir is injected into the residual papillomas, leaving the anterior and posterior commissures intact on purpose. This procedure avoids the formation of anterior synechiae of the vocal cords or of posterior glottal stenosis. The ultimate objective is to avoid synechia formation. When the disease is limited to the larynx, an optimal quality of the voice rather than the total resection of all papillomas, should be prioritized [1].

Considering the unpredictable course of the disease and the possible improvement at the time of puberty, limiting the number of debulking sessions and carefully removing papillomas is essential for preventing scar sequels [1].

Prevention

Two vaccines against HPV have been developed to prevent cervical and uterine cancer caused by HPV. These vaccines are Cervarix ® (bivalent, with virus-like particle combination based on HPV-16 and HPV-18) and Gardasil ® (quadrivalent, with virus-like combination also based on HPV-6 and HPV-11) [11, 13]. Important randomized clinical trials have demonstrated that the quadrivalent vaccine is highly effective in preventing the genital infection and cervical dysplasia associated with HPV types 6, 11, 16 and 18, and genital condilomas in women not previously infected by HPV. The bivalent vaccine has also been effective in the prevention of cervical dysplasia but does not protect against types 6 and 11 infections. Therefore, no impact on the incidence of RRP is expected [13].

The best hope lies in the quadrivalent vaccine against HPV subtypes 6, 11, 16 and 18. Vaccination of both men and women before starting an active sex life promises to remarkably reduce disease incidence [27, 28].

Additional studies have assessed safety and immunogenicity persistence in both male and female children. The vaccine is often well tolerated, inducing an anti-HPV serological response both in boys and girls, lasting for at least 3.5 years post-term after vaccination schedule; therefore, booster doses of the vaccine do not seem to be necessary [13].

If the vaccine succeeds in being effective in reducing the incidence of HPV-related cervical and vaginal disease, then RRP incidence could also be reduced or eradicated in the future.

Furthermore, the vaccine induces antibodies that could pass through the placenta, thus providing some benefits against HPV-infection [29]. Moreover, there are some other studies that highlight the therapeutic value of the quadrivalent vaccine [30, 31].

CONCLUSION

Dysphonia is a tell-tale sign that is often ignored by parents, patients and even by physicians. It is an alarm signal in children, which is not as important as in adults, since laryngeal cancer is rare in childhood. In addition, as the examination of the larynx may be complicated and difficult, most often the study is postponed without having an accurate diagnosis. An early recognition of voice disorders as well as an evaluation of the airway in all newborns, infants and children experiencing persistent hoarseness is vital to establish a firm diagnosis and an adequate treatment.

RRP can be suspected if a child experiences progressive dysphonia with no periods of normal voice. Since RRP tends to relapse, has an unpredictable clinical course and poses the risk of malignant transformation, a close follow-up of the patient suffering from laryngeal papillomatosis and viral typification of the lesions are of vital importance. We strongly recommend to perform a biopsy on all patients with papillomatosis to determine the histological features of the lesions. Extralaryngeal dissemination worsens disease prognosis.

References

[1] Monnier P. Recurrent respiratory papillomatosis. In: Monnier P, editor. Pediatric airway surgery. Management of laryngotracheal stenosis in infants and children. *Springer*, Switzerland; 2011:220-7.

[2] Sánchez de Losada F. Papilomatosis laríngea recurrente. In: Sih T, Chinski A, et al. editors. VI Manual de Otorrinolaringología pediátrica de la IAPO; 2008: 96-8.

[3] Fusconi M, Grasso M, Greco A, Gallo A, Campo F, Remacle M, Turchetta R, Pagliuca G, De Vincentiis M. Recurrent respiratory papillomatosis by HPV: review of the literature and update on the use of cidofovir. *Acta Otorhinolaryngol. Ital. 2014*; 34(6):375-81.

[4] Marsico M, Mehta V, Chastek B, Liaw KL, Derkay C. Estimating the incidence and prevalence of juvenile onset recurrent respiratory papillomatosis in publicly and privately insured claims databases in the United States. *Sex Transm. Dis.* 2014; 41(5):300-5.

[5] Rodríguez H, Cuestas G, Roques M, Rodríguez D´Aquila JA. Estridores laríngeos. In: Sih T, Chisnki A, et al. editors. XII IAPO Manual de Otorrinolaringología Pediátrica de la IAPO. Gráfica Forma Certa, San Pablo, Brasil; 2014: 95-128.

[6] Rodríguez H, Cuestas G. Papilomatosis laríngea y voz. In: Rodríguez H, editor. VII Manual de la asociación argentina de ORL y fonoaudiología pediátrica. *Disfonías infantiles*; 2014: 104-6.

[7] Rodríguez V, Michalski D. Papilomatosis laríngea infantil. *Revista FASO* 2010; 17: 16-22.

[8] Herrera Martínez E, Aguilar Sánchez J, Torres Poveda K, Madrid Marina V. Tipificación del virus del papiloma humano en lesiones del epitelio respiratorio. *An Orl. Mex* .2013; 58: 207-11.

[9] Omland T, Akre H, Lie KA, Jebsen P, Sandvik L, Brøndbo K. Risk factors for aggressive recurrent respiratory papillomatosis in adults and juveniles. *PLoS One* 2014; 9 (11):e113584.

[10] Richardson MA, Faust RA. Papilomatosis respiratoria recurrente. In: Suarez C, Gil Carcedo LM, et al. editors. Tratado de Otorrinolaringología y Cirugía de Cabeza y Cuello. Editorial Médica Panamericana, Buenos Aires – Madrid; 2008: 2601-7.

[11] Carifi M, Napolitano D, Morandi M, Dall´Ollio D. Recurrent respiratory papillomatosis: current and future perspectives. *Ther. Clin. Risk Manag.* 2015:11: 731-8.

[12] Measso do Bonfim C, Simão Sobrinho J, Lacerda Nogueira R, Salgado Kupper D, Cardoso Pereira Valera F, Lacerda Nogueira M, Villa LL, Rahal P, Sichero L. Differences in transcriptional activity of human papillomavirus type 6 molecular variants in recurrent respiratory papillomatosis. *PLoS One* 2015; 10(7):e0132325.

[13] Sahba Sedaghat N. Papilomatosis respiratoria recurrente y el rol de la vacunación antiVPH. *Rev. Otorrinolaringol. Cir. Cabeza Cuello* 2013; 73(1): 89-93.

[14] Wang J, Han DM, Ma LJ, Ye JY, Xiao Y, Yang QW. Risk factors of juvenile onset recurrent respiratory papillomatosis in the lower respiratory tract. *Chin. Med. J. (Engl)* 2012; 125(19):3496-9.

[15] Derkay CS, Volsky PG, Rosen CA, Pransky SM, McMurray JS, Chadha NK, Froehlich P. Current use of intralesional cidofovir for recurrent respiratory papillomatosis. *Laryngoscope* 2013; 123(3):705-12.

[16] Pransky ST, Albright MA, Magit AE. Long term follow up of pediatric recurrent respiratory papillomatosis managed with intralesional cidofovir. *Laryngoscope* 2003; 113(9):1583-7.

[17] Gomes Avelino M, Teixeira Zaiden T, Oliveira Gomes R. Surgical treatment and adjuvant therapies of recurrent respiratory papillomatosis. *Braz. J. Otorhinolaryngol.* 2013; 79(5):636-42.

[18] Sidell DR, Nassar M, Cotton RT, Zeitels SM, de Alarcon A. High-dose sublesional bevacizumab (avastin) for pediatric recurrent respiratory papillomatosis. *Ann. Otol. Rhinol. Laryngol.* 2014; 123(3):214-21.

[19] Zeitels SM, Barbu AM, Landau-Zemer T, Lopez-Guerra G, Burns JA, Friedman AD, Freeman MW, Halvorsen YD, Hillman RE. Local injection of bevacizumab (Avastin) and angiolytic KTP laser treatment of recurrent respiratory papillomatosis of the vocal folds: a prospective study. *Ann. Otol. Rhinol. Laryngol.* 2011; 120(10):627-34.

[20] Best SR, Friedman AD, Landau-Zemer T, Barbu AM, Burns JA, Freeman MW, Halvorsen YD, Hillman RE, Zeitels SM. Safety and dosing of bevacizumab (avastin) for the treatment of recurrent respiratory papillomatosis. *Ann. Otol. Rhinol. Laryngol.* 2012; 121(9):587-93.

[21] Rangel-Chávez JJ, Espinosa-Martínez C, Rangel-Audelo R. Aplicación de bevacizumab (Avastin®) en papiloma recurrente sin uso de láser KTP. *An Orl. Mex.* 2015; 60:109-13.

[22] Rogers DJ, Ojha S, Maurer R, Hartnick CJ. Use of adjuvant intralesional bevacizumb for aggressive respiratory papillomatosis in children. *JAMA Otolaryngol. Head Neck Surg.* 2013; 139(5):496-501.

[23] Nagel S, Busch C, Blankenburg T, Schütte W. Treatment of respiratory papillomatosis--a case report on systemic treatment with bevacizumab [Article in German]. *Pneumologie* 2009; 63(7):387-9.

[24] Mohr M, Schliemann C, Biernann C, Schmidt LH, Kessler T, Schmidt J, Wiebe K, Müller KM, Hoffmann TK, Groll AH, Werner C, Kessler C, Wiewrodt R, Rudack C, Berdel WE. Rapid response to systemic bevacizumab therapy in recurrent respiratory papillomatosis. *Oncol. Lett.* 2014; 8(5):1912-8.

[25] Woo P. Benign tumors. In: Woo P, editor. Stroboscopy. Plural Publishing, Inc, United Kingdom; 2010: 305-12.

[26] Willging JP. Laryngeal neoplasms. In: Myers III Ch, Cotton R, et al, editors. The pediatric airway. An interdisciplinary approach. JB Lippincott Company, Philadelphia; 1995: 263-76.

[27] Venkatesan NN, Pine HS, Underbrink MP. Recurrent respiratory papillomatosis. *Otolaryngol. Clin. North. Am.* 2012; 45(3):671-94.

[28] Donne AJ, Clarke R. Recurrent respiratory papillomatosis: an uncommon but potentially devastating effect of human papillomavirus in children. *Int. J. STD AIDS* 2010; 21(6):381-5.

[29] Matys K, Mallary S, Bautista O, Vuocolo S, Manalastas R, Pitisuttithum P, Saah A. Mother-infant transfer of anti-human papillomavirus (HPV) antibodies following vaccination with the quadrivalent HPV (type 6/11/16/18) virus-like particle vaccine. *Clin. Vaccine Immunol.* 2012; 19(6):881-5.

[30] Mudry P. Recurrent respiratory papillomatosis (RRP) - succesful treatment with HPV vaccination. *Arch. Dis. Child* 2012.

[31] Hamsikova E. Recurrent respiratory papillomatosis (RRP) and HPV vaccination. *IPC Berlin* 2011.

In: Voice Disorders
Editor: Derrick Welch
ISBN: 978-1-63484-413-0

Chapter 3

PEDIATRIC VOICE THERAPY: BIG CHALLENGE WITH LITTLE PEOPLE

Susana Vaz-Freitas*[1,*], *SLP, MSc, PhD, and Pedro Melo Pestana*[2], *SLP
[1]Speech Therapy Department of Otolaryngology Service, Centro Hospitalar do Porto, Porto, Portugal
[2]PMP Terapia, Esposende, Portugal

ABSTRACT

Dysphonia is present in a growing number of children, resulting in a negative impact on social interaction and academic proficiency. Although some laryngeal lesions or voice disorders can be found more frequently in children, its physiopathology as well as its functional outcomes are not significantly different from those found in adults. Besides the well known anatomic and physiological differences, the great challenge approaching childhood dysphonia lies in their peculiar social and behavioral characteristics.

This chapter aims to present the latest investigation results related to Speech and Language Pathology intervention in childhood dysphonia. Voice development is described. Furthermore, the authors present assessment protocols and therapeutic approaches commonly used in voice disorders within the pediatric population. Early identification and awareness improvement among family and school settings play a key role

* Email: svazfreitas@gmail.com.

in voice therapy outcomes. Finally, the authors propose a structured intervention protocol and a summary table presenting the most common laryngeal disorders and their characteristics in childhood dysphonia.

Keywords: childhood dysphonia, assessment, identification, intervention, quality of life

1. Introduction

The number of cases of childhood or pediatric dysphonia has been increasing, as well as the consequent interest and study of the topic and the characterization of the factors that underlie its pathogenesis (Angelillo et al., 2008). There are few studies that prove and detail this statement.

Dysphonia occurs when a different anatomical, physiological and functional criteria are combined resulting from a vocal pattern that deviates from the expected for age and gender. So, it is possible to deal with cases where there is a diagnosed anatomical change, but the speaker does not recognize it as impacting in different settings of voice use; or else that denotes difficulties in the use of voice in a given situation, but without any diagnosed evidence of laryngeal disorder or vocal tract.

The diagnosis of dysphonia or voice quality disorder is usually done when the misuses and abuses have caused structural changes in the vocal folds (Angelillo et al., 2008). The importance of assessing the child according to spontaneous and connected speech has been already demonstrated (Sederholm, 1996c). Thus, this author concluded that connected speech is perceived as containing more breaks, significantly more hoarse but less unstable compared to sustained vowels, commonly used in most vocal assessment protocols.

The first, large and significant prospective study on the prevalence of dysphonia in childhood was made by Carding et al., (2006) through the analysis of a large cohort (7389) of children with 8 years old. The prevalence of pediatric voice disorders was 6%. During childhood, the age group that presents a greater representation of dysphonia is between 8 and 14 proven by a prevalence of 59.6% (Angelillo et al., 2008). Other research confirms that among patients with dysphonia, 17.2% are aged between 2 and 16 (Angelillo et al., 2008).

Concerning gender distribution, boys are more prevalent than girls, although this trend is mostly evident up to ten years old (Carding et al., 2006). This can be explained due to the personality characteristics of boys, as well as the social and physical activities that are developed by boys, involving an excessive and inappropriate use of voice. Unlike adult patients with dysphonia, in children boys are more susceptible to present it (57%).

Authors found that 90.3% of children with vocal fold pathologies show lesions that are, in descending order: irregularity between the anterior and middle third of the vocal folds (59.9%); vocal fold nodules (24.95%) and edema (5.5%) (Angelillo et al., 2008).

2. The Voice in Childhood: Little Big Differences

2.1. Anatomical and Physiological Peculiarities of Children's Larynx

The anatomy and physiological behavior of the larynx change gradually with age.

In newborns, the lower edge of the cricoid is located between the 3rd and 4th cervical vertebrae. Until two years old, it reaches the inferior part of C5 and at the age of five, it can be found at C6 middle part. At 15 years old, the inferior part of the cricoid is between C6 and C7. As age increases, the larynx continues to descend until it reaches the inferior part of C7 (Sederholm, 1996a).

Up to ten years of age there is no difference in the length of the vocal folds between genders. From the age of fifteen a great difference can be found, with an increased growth of the vocal fold length in boys (Sederholm, 1996a).

The histology of the vocal fold also varies with age. The newborn has no vocal ligament and the whole lamina propria is uniform. The differentiation begins between six and twelve years old and at fifteen three distinct layers are found (Gray, Hirano and Sato, 1993 cit. In Sederholm, 1996a). According to these authors the complete development of intrinsic laryngeal muscles is only reached around 25 years old.

2.2. Voice Development: Considerations around Speech and Singing in Children

According to the pitch, the vocal range in non-singing children with normal voice quality is around 24 semitones (st). Maximum phonation time of alveolar fricatives and the s/z coefficient changes according to the age (cf. Table 1).

In children with chronic dysphonia pitch range average is 22 st. In mutational voices it is 29 st; in cases with glottal gap is 27 st, and in children with vocal fold nodules is 19 st. The average dynamic range of sound pressure level varies between 22.8 and 21.4 dB (McAllister, Sederholm, Sundberg, & Gramming, 1994).

Table 1. Maximum phonation time (MPT) and s/z coefficient, Tait et al., (1980) cit. In McNeil (1997)

Gender	Age	MPT of/s/		MPT of/z/		s/z coefficient	
		Average	Amplitude	Average	Amplitude	Average	Amplitude
Boys	5	7.9	5.4 - 9.8	8.6	6.6 - 13.0	0.92	0,82- 1,08
	7	9.3	7.4 - 12.5	13.2	9.2 - 19.6	0.7	0.52 - 0.97
	9	16.7	7.1 - 44.0	18.1	10.1 - 33.1	0.92	0.41 - 2.67
Girls	5	8.3	4.8 - 18.3	10	5.2 - 16.0	0.83	0.50 - 1.14
	7	10.2	7.3 - 16.0	13.1	9.1 - 20.0	0.78	0.51 - 1.10
	9	14.4	9.3 - 20.9	15.8	8.5 - 24.2	0.91	0.75 - 1.26

Regular vocal training undoubtedly improves children's voice abilities. According to Fuchs et al. (2009), those that go under training have the following modified characteristics:

- The higher the voice demand and training, the greater perception and conscious control of the voice. It is also known that as the training increases, voice range and tessitura becomes wider;
- Besides controlling their voice more consciously, boys have higher values of maximum phonation time, maximum loudness range and greater ability to vary pitch and loudness;

Regular voice training not only has the intention to increase singing skills, but also assumes a preventive role from the clinical standpoint (Fuchs et al., 2009; Simões, 2008).

2.3. Early Detection and Risk Factors

The parents' awareness in primary health services is crucial. Carding et al. (2006) state that there is a small percentage of parents who, unlike clinicians, believe that children never had a voice alteration. In clinical voice practice, parents often find that the voice of their children have frequent moments of hoarseness or strain - however, usually, they don't value those signs.

Parents describe the dysphonic voice of their children as "much stronger, less clear, less stable and more sensitive to changes" relating to their peers (Sederholm, McAllister, Dalkvist & Sundberg, 1995).

The detection of this condition during pediatric age is more likely if parents have already had another son for comparison (Carding et al., 2006).

Here we present a collection of risk factors and the pathogenesis of childhood dysphonia, leading to strenuous use of voice:

- Have, at least, an older or younger sibling (89%) (Carding et al., 2006)
- Presence of older brothers in the family (Carding et al., 2006)
- Aggressive and hyperactive behavior (83%), where the child uses his voice to assert themselves (Angelillo et al., 2008)
- Family history of the same disorder (30%), leading to a imitation pattern (Angelillo et al., 2008)
- Large families with more than two children, representing 65% of cases (to get attention) (Angelillo et al.2008)
- Using the voice intensively (Bhattarai, 2010; Boseley, Cunningham, Volk, & Hartnick, 2006; Connor et al, 2008; Roy, Holt, Redmond, & Muntz, 2007; Sederholm, 1996b)
- Children who are more talkative than their pairs (Sederholm, 1996b)

It is also known that older children are more likely to imitate other voices, for instance, it is common among boys to imitate the hoarse voice of rock singers (Fuchs et al., 2009) or the noise of machines and transports, while playing.

Children with siblings are more likely to develop dysphonia and it can be justified due to the great vocal demands, to the competition for the speech turn and to the need to overlap the surrounding noise (Carding et al., 2006).

Against some myths, we present some data evidenced by Carding et al., (2006). His team showed that the following are not considered as risk factors: high level of noise at home, to have asthma, have had otitis media or have undergone adenoidectomy or tonsillectomy. These results contradict what parents considered as potential causal factors. It should be noted that in the presence of the listed conditions, a transitory period of voice disorder can exist (e.g., in the immediate post-operative).

3. From Detection to Diagnosis: What to Expect?

3.1. The Most Common Functional Diagnostics

Attached to this chapter a table can be found including the organic and functional conditions that lead, commonly, to a voice change and its main features (Appendix II).

Vocal nodules are the most common lesions of the vocal folds in children as a result of vocal abuse and glottal hyper function. Although there is some consistency, its progression is variable, taking into account some factors such as age, gender and other parameters. When the vocal nodules appear in childhood, its remission in post-pubertal stage of boys is more often than girls (De Bodt et al., 2007). This does not mean that there are no laryngeal or vocal changes as minimal changes can persist, such as glottal gap and edema. Often, when a glottal gap is present, there is an increase of the average amount of air that results in effective phonation; furthermore, the mass lesions predict an increase of subglottic pressure needed to start vibration (which may or may not result in glottal gap).

It should be noted that a negative impact in social and academic participation of these children can exist, dependent on: the type of vocal disorder - congenital or acquired; the severity of voice alteration; the child's and peers' reaction; the reaction/attitude of parents and caregivers.

The severity of lesions depends on compensatory strategies already adopted by the subject - so, the longer is the dysphonia installation time, the more likely the child tries to compensate the vocal difficulties and keeps a modified speaking pattern worsening the disorder.

3.2. Puberphonia: A General Rule

Several milestones mark the children’s normal development. Although voice changes occur in different age ranks between genders (men: 13-15 years; girls: 9-16 years), they have similar impact on the subject. Puberty is noted by rapid muscle development, growth in height and weight (Seikel, King, & Drumright, 2010).

Obviously, the structures involved in phonation are no exception. The thyroid cartilage and thyroarytenoid muscle are the structures that have higher growth, not only but mainly in boys (Seikel, King & Drumright, 2010).

Those structural changes alter vocal physiology as well, with greater impact on boys. The breaks in pitch are the most frequent vocal behaviors observed during this phase, resulting from a combination of tissue change and the attempt to control this change in the fundamental frequency of the voice.

Various names are used in order to categorize normal or deviant voice during this stage.

Puberphonia can be defined as the continuous use of children's vocal characteristics during the period of body growth at puberty. Thus, there is a clear discrepancy between a childhood voice and a body that is coming closer and closer to adulthood. The high pitch and its inherent breaks are the most noticeable features, especially in boys (Seikel, King & Drumright, 2010).

Regarding Speech and Language Pathology intervention, during adolescence there is a strategy that seems to result in reducing the negative impact on social life: if the voice therapy is done during the summer holidays, school mates will not notice the results so immediately, which decreases the likelihood of comments or speculation.

4. Intervention: Difficult Decision-Making

To define the term "normal voice" is difficult and a nonconsensual task. The boundaries between normal voice and dysphonia are also difficult to establish. To these two variables it is impossible not to add another: when should we consider dysphonia?

As was demonstrated in this review, the child is faced with the challenge of a number of typical development events, whether the child is normal or not. Their social and behavioral characteristics are also an important factor to take into account.

Note that whenever a child is referred, the child must be assessed. Regarding clinical setting - according to the Phoniatry Committee of the European Laryngological Society (ELS) - voice assessment must include the collection of information through: (1) clinical history or clinical interview; (2) assessment of laryngeal physiology (indirect laryngoscopy and/or endoscopy and/or stroboscopic and/or electroglottography, among others); (3) audio perceptual assessment; (4) Functional evaluation (aerodynamic and musculoskeletal assessment); (5) acoustic analysis; and (6) self-assessment of voice impact in psychosocial domain (Dejonckere et al., 2001).

However, major dilemmas can exist affecting decision-making regarding cases of childhood dysphonia, namely: shall we intervene? When? With whom? How; what kind of therapy shall we choose? What benefits will this intervention bring?

For the authors of this chapter, if any doubt exists to consider a voice as dysphonic, its impact on a person's quality of life data must be collected, including the voice capacity to meet the challenges that the child undergoes.

The aim of the next few paragraphs is to reiterate a philosophy of thought that the authors consider to be the most appropriate facing cases of childhood dysphonia, rather than convey theoretical content.

4.1. From Therapeutic Goal to Generalization

Before anything, the speech and language pathologist must be aware of the laryngeal physical condition of that particular child, as well as the state of other organs involved in speech. This procedure must be done by the ENT specialist and the images and report must be delivered to the speech and language pathologist as complete as possible. Considerations regarding the mucosal wave, type of glottal occlusion and presence of mass lesions must be expected. The use of audio-visual media is, nowadays, easy and basic. If there is an indication for surgery, speech therapy should be included in pre- and post-surgery (Marsal & Vila, 2005) in order to ensure adequate post-operative results.

According to Azevedo (2010) voice therapy must be done fulfilling the following order: orientation of those involved in the process; vocal hygiene; vocal psychodynamics; voice training itself. This model follows what is recommended by Behlau et al. (2001), which is traditionally identified as the Global Method.

Based on these ordered phases, an intervention protocol was elaborated. Authors supported their reasoning on the most recent studies with a high level of evidence (see Appendix I). This protocol is compiled from some cited materials and professional experience of the authors.

At the *orientation* stage (Phase I), the clinician must convey to the child, caregivers and involved educational team (parents, teachers, peers ...) basic concepts of voice anatomy and physiology as well as pathophysiology of dysphonia. Prognosis, type of approach, duration of therapy and discharge criteria shall be discussed during this stage (Azevedo, 2010). These must be the first goals of the clinician, right after the assessment. It is important to remember that all the people involved in the process should be part of decision making: since the type of approach until discharge. Still, the clinician must be able to present all the information in a comprehensive but simplified manner, always depending on the person he is interacting with (Carding et al., 2006).

It is very important to have materials adapted to children with interactive potential and representativeness of the shared information (see Table 2). We recommend the use of current cartoon characters, customized programs/software similar to those available nowadays. Material or therapy resources made with the child's participation are more meaningful.

Changes to a child's routine must be clarified and are supported in motivation. Children motivation will be achieved if the clinician knows how to argue meaningfully; interesting moments and activities to the child must be evoked so they can be immediately applicable in their daily lives (eg, how would you call your friend in the playground?).

Table 2. Examples of funny images used in Phase I

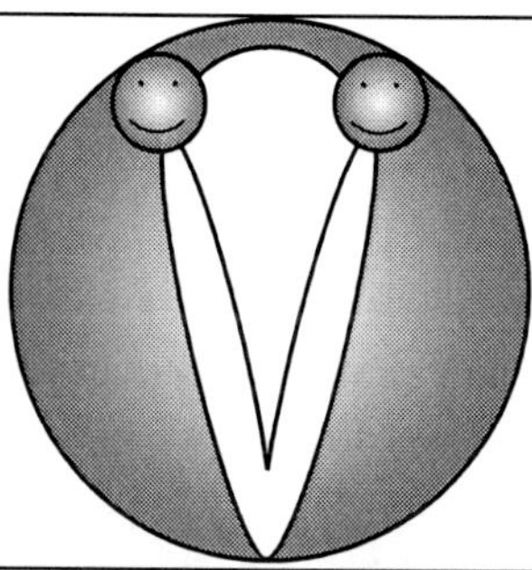	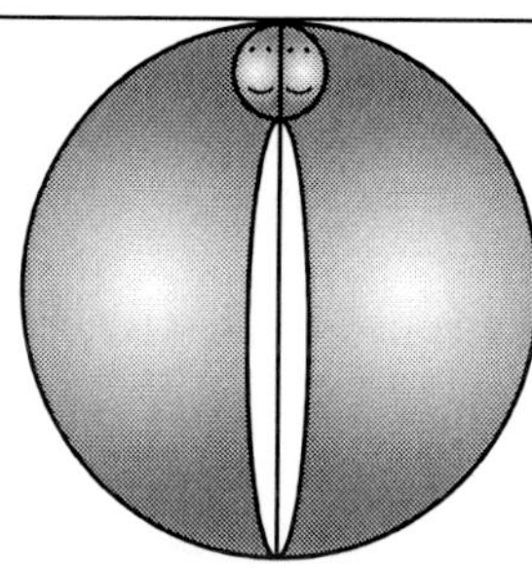
a) glottis in abduction / breathing	b) glottis in adduction / phonation
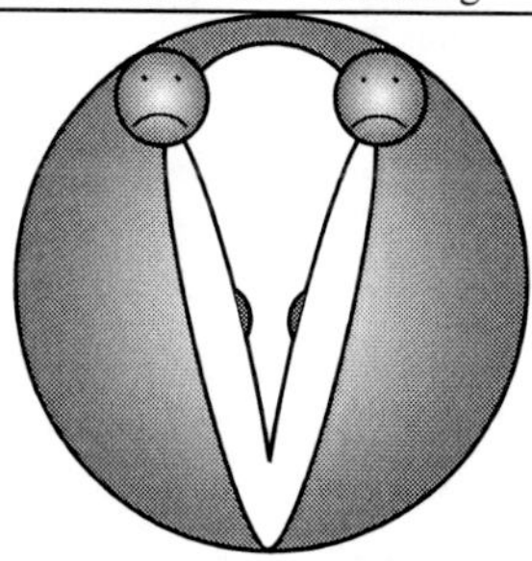	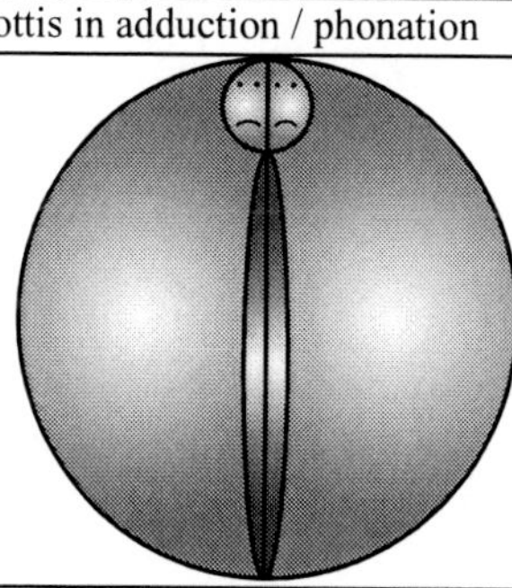
c) with bilateral vocal fold nodules	d) glottis in hyper function and/or oedema

The inclusion in therapy of parents and teachers/educators is inevitable, because they are who spend more time with the child. It may be useful in the following situations: identifying moments or behaviors that promote the voice disorder; providing data about the interaction of the child with peers and family; they are another therapy agent, especially useful in monitoring the progression of dysphonia, implementation strategies and controlling/restricting vocal abuses that occur in extra-therapy settings.

The health and vocal hygiene issue (Phase II) is, undoubtedly, very important. As has been already demonstrated, the etiology of most pediatric dysphonia is - directly or indirectly - vocal misuse and abusive behaviors (see Table 1 - Risk factors).

Vocal attitude changes proposed by the clinician can be counterproductive. For example, the clinician recommends cessation of the use of a loud voice during physical activity (e.g., soccer, basketball, hockey, karate). The clinician can be almost certain that this was the behavior that led to the vocal nodules, but the elimination of this child activity may not imply the immediate disappearance of lesions.

Careful identification of misuse and abusive vocal behaviors should be made, but not overvalued. The negative reinforcement and activities deprivation can lead to compromising effects regarding motivation and therapy success.

According to Marsal & Vila (2005) the primary therapy goal should be the child's awareness about dysphonia, which is a central part of vocal psychodynamics (Phase III). Azevedo (2010) proposes playful activities for vocal psychodynamics. All have a cognitive based intervention and are used in order to increase the vocal self-awareness. For example, to classify other voice`s by assigning characteristics (emotions, gender, age, etc.) in given speech samples. The discussion about basic communication rules may have a very positive influence on changing the child's, caregivers and teachers/educators attitudes.

The changes in the child's voice are achieved by increasing the "auditory attention, discrimination, perception and the ability to assimilate concepts involved in this process" (Azevedo, 2010). The author proposes the use of TV cartoon clips as an intervention resource.

Therapy methods and techniques, *per se* (Stage IV) are not that different from those used for adults. The big difference is the intensity and frequency in which they are applied/prescribed and, fundamentally, the way they are presented, explained and repeated by and to the child. There is a consensus that the intervention in childhood dysphonia must be based, mainly, in the indirect approach. Thus, the intensity of this stage doesn't play the major role and will be smaller than with adults.

4.2. Auto-Perception of Voice in Children

The development of a treatment plan should always take into account some intervention principles adapted to the child (Marsal & Vila, 2005). The great difference between the child and the adult with dysphonia is the past experience. The awareness that a child may have about his disordered voice quality is little or none, as he didn't have much time with the other standard. On the other hand, adult perceives dysphonia more easily, since the voice was constant until the establishment of the onset of the disorder. This is the reason for auditory discrimination training. The child could, for example, classify voices according to gender, age, quality, pitch, loudness, etc. (Azevedo, 2010; Marsal & Vila, 2005). The use of speech samples of cartoon characters is suggested, with adequate and inadequate vocal patterns.

Relaxation, posture and breathing are the intervention components that follow, with the premise that voice is movement (Azevedo, 2010; Marsal & Vila, 2005; Seikel et al., 2010).

Note that after completion of the listed skills, a direct approach is required as much as possible. The selection of voice methods and techniques should be made based on organic or functional etiology of the child dysphonia, just as with an adult. The difficulty is in presentation of the techniques to the child - based on their understanding, attention and development stage.

4.3. Adapted Available Resources

In Portugal and Portuguese language there are few resources for voice therapy, especially for children intervention. It is common that Speech and Language Pathologists build their own intervention materials, while the access to those that have been published is difficult.

To help on the execution of techniques or vocal exercises, there is some playful software, which gives visual feedback of different voice parameters (pitch, loudness, voicing, etc.). Based on goals, clinician can select these activities. Table 3 presents a list of those that are used the most.

Another available resource are printed books written by Speech Pathologists, filled with therapy activities linked to the different stages of the voice recovery process (Behlau et al., 1997; Cotes, 1997; Martins, sd; Gasparini et al., 2006; Melo, Caeiro and Lavra, 2006; Muniz, 2010).

Table 3. Software and commercial company

Software Name	Company
Voice Games	KayPentax
VoxGames - Therapy Voice	CTS Hardware
Voice games (opensource)	Digital Speech Processing Laboratory at UNICAMP
Dr. Speech - Voice Therapy	Tiger DRS, Inc.

5. Dysphonia: The Impact on Children's Quality of Life

The impact of dysphonia on the child's quality of life is big, as can be confirmed below. Emotional issues are more exacerbated in adolescence, due to changes in personality and body appearance. Thus, the comparison between peers will have a greater impact on them. This is a mandatory parameter to be assessed in children with dysphonia. Formally or informally, this topic has to be approached to know child and parent perception regarding the impact of the clinical condition. While doing this, the clinician can also infer about child and caregivers motivation to recovery. There are quite a few protocols to collect this kind of information: *Pediatric Voice Outcome Survey* (Hartnick, 2002); the *Pediatric Voice-Related Quality-of-Life Survey* into English (Boseley et al., 2006); the *Pediatric Voice Handicap Index* (pVHI) into English (Zur et al, 2007) and Italian (Schindler et al., 2007). The Pediatric Voice Symptom Questionnaire (Verduyckt, Morsomme and Remacle, 2012) includes a version for the child and one for parents/caregivers.

The main feelings associated with dysphonia in children and parents are sadness, anxiety, frustration and shame. Children are often reported as having a different voice comparing to peers and that difference is also commented by other people. Furthermore, the feeling of "dry mouth" associated with the use of voice is usually reported, which is easily surpassed with water intake (Connor et al., 2008). In children with dysphonia between 2 and 4 years old it is common to find teachers/caregivers asking the child to be quieter and not to use much voice. Frustration and behavioral problems are reinforced due to the difficulty of being heard (Connor et al., 2008). Between 5 and 7 years old the most affected area is the physical one, complaining of "running out of air" and "difficulty initiating a voice effortlessly"; still, periods of aphonia are also reported as "run out of voice." It is still quite common at this age that adults ask the child to speak with less intensity than usual. Not so common but still important, children can refer the feeling of "burned throat" (Connor et al., 2008).

Between 8 and 12 years old, the most affected areas are the physical and social/functional. The main concerns are "lost their voice," "run out of air" and "dry mouth" associated with the use of voice. It remains frequent the feeling of "burning throat." Regarding second area, friends and colleagues usually make questions about the lesion or vocal condition. Commonly, they are embarrassing and increase anxiety and fear during pre-teen stage, which leads to a decrease of their participation, for instance, in the classroom (e.g., reading activity to the class). Humiliation is, sometimes, more frequently from those that are not expected to (eg. teachers or other people that do not know them) (Connor et al., 2008). In the age rank of 13 to 18 years old, the most affected areas are usually physical and emotional. From the physical standpoint, the following problems are reported: "inability to be heard," "dry mouth," "difficulty in singing voice" and "increased effort to speak." Dysphonia interferes a lot with their activities. Regarding emotional domain, the fear of not being able to speak is reported, as well as the frustration of being left out in the activities. In social/functional domains, teenagers are is afraid that others will laugh when the voice is produced with change. It should be noted that they "are already tired of answering questions about their voice quality" (Connor et al., 2008).

CONCLUSION

Speech Language Pathology with pediatric dysphonia is increasingly common and a primary concern is required: a constant adjustment to the comprehension and attention skills is needed and must include changes in daily life outside the therapy room. Adherence to therapy can and should be enhanced by the degree of empathy established between the professional and the child, as well as the use of appealing materials to present the intervention goals. More than in any other age group, the Speech Pathologist has to prove his technical and scientific knowledge as well as being able to adapt it to this very special type of clients.

APPENDIX I. BASICS FOR THERAPY IN CHILDHOOD DYSPHONIA

The following protocol is intended to be the basis for a therapy plan in this field. It should not, at any time, replace clinical reasoning, adjustment to particularities of each child or laryngeal specific condition. The number of sessions is only an estimate, based on the authors' experience. It should be mentioned that although presenting a hierarchy of objectives in the different stages of intervention, it does not mean that an earlier stage is not repeated furthermore

Stages (Number of Appointments)	Procedures (the clinician should be able to ...)	Specific goals for the child/family (the child/family should be able to...)
STAGE 1: Instructions to therapy participants (1st and 2nd appointment)	1.1 Collect personal and clinical data 1.2 Collect of information relatied to the environmental conditions of the vocal use 1.3 Collect data on interaction of children with peers and family 1.4 Audio perceptual and acoustic assessment 1.5 Assessment of the auto perception of the impact of dysphonia in quality of life 1.6 Present basics of voice production 1.7 Present basics of dysphonia 1.8 Prognosis discussion 1.9 Discussion of the therapy approach 1.10 Discussion of the expected time for therapy 1.11 Discussion of the therapy discharge criteria	1.1 Provide relevant data on their personal, family, academic and clinical life (child and family) 1.2 Provide relevant data about daily vocal use (child and family) 1.3 Provide relevant data about child-adult and child-peers voice interaction 1.4 Cooperate in the audio perceptual and acoustic assessment (child) 1.5 Cooperate in the auto perception of the impact of dysphonia in quality of life assessment (child and family) 1.6 Summarize the anatomy and physiology of speech production (child and family) 1.7 Summarize the pathophysiology of that specific vocal lesion (child and family) 1.8 Accept the prognosis established by the clinician (child and family) 1.9 Engage in decisions regarding the intervention plan (child and family) 1.10 Accept clinician's decision regarding the time for effective intervention (child and family) 1.11 Define, together with the clinician, the therapy discharge criteria

<table>
<tr><td>STAGE 2: Vocal Health
(3rd and 4th appointment)</td><td>2.1 Inform about vocal misuses and abuses
2.2 Justify each change needed to control the vocal misuse and abuse
2.3 Identify traumatic vocal behaviors
2.4 Present alternatives to traumatic vocal behaviors
2.5 Advise about restriction/elimination of traumatic vocal behaviors</td><td>2.1 Summarize behaviors of vocal abuse and misuse identifying them in their reality (child)
2.2 Explain the need to fullfil rules of vocal health (child and family)
2.3 Identify and define traumatic vocal behaviors (child and family)
2.4 Contribute with alternatives to the traumatic vocal behaviors (family and child)
2.5 Reduce/eliminate selected traumatic vocal behaviors (child)</td></tr>
<tr><td>STAGE 3: Vocal Psychodynamic
(5th to 7th appointment - with the children and their privileged communicative peers)</td><td>3.1 Present different auditory stimuli with antagonistic features: loudness, pitch, duration (auditory discrimination)
3.2 Inform about the impact that different postures have in voice production (posture and verticality)
3.3 Present the interdependence of vocal tract elements during voice production (voice preparation)</td><td>3.1.1 Listen and identify noises and sounds with/without visual support
3.1.2 Listen and identify sound situations with/without visual support. 3.1.3 Discriminate and classify sounds: loudness, pitch, duration
3.2.1 Identify the correct horizontal and vertical body positioning
3.2.2 Reorder the correct support and verticality starting from different positions
3.2.3 List different postures in daily activities with vocal use and its impact on voice quality
3.3.1 Identify phono-articulatory and resonance structures
3.3.2 Recognize that voice propagates along the vocal tract (action of phono-articulatory and resonance structures)
3.3.2 List the movement possibilities of speech and resonance structures
3.3.3 Identify different vocal qualities resulting from vocal tract adjustments
3.3.4 Identify phonation with and without glottal attacks</td></tr>
<tr><td>STAGE 4: Vocal Training
(7th to 13th appointment)</td><td colspan="2">Traditional methods and techniques should be used as much as possible. Its selection depends on larynx condition and underlying voice adjustments, as in the adult. Its use should account child's skills and never miss the playful standpoint.</td></tr>
</table>

Appendix II. Most Common Laryngeal Pathologies in Pediatric Age and Its Vocal Characteristics

(Verdolini et al., 2005; Mitchell and Pereira, 2009; Graham, Scadding and Bull, 2007; Angelillo et al., 2008) When referring to traumatic vocal behavior, authors assume it as "excessive or inadequate voice use that promotes dysphonia." Example: imitation sound of animals or toys, cheerleading, singing without training or technique, screaming, voice use in noisy environments, etc.

Classification (Lesion or Disorder)	Organic and Functional Disorders	Causes/Associated Behaviors	Aerodynamic and acoustic characteristics	Observations
Vocal Nodules (78% of the chronic pediatric dysphonia)	Benign mass lesion, bilateral, not always symmetric Localized on the vocal fold lamina propria, between the anterior third and the two posterior thirds Incomplete glottal closure – hourglass-shape configuration	Traumatic vocal behavior Excessive voice use, strained Shouting Personality – outgoing Dehydration Allergies Dry environments Pharyngo-Esophageal Reflux	Roughness and Breathiness Phono-asthenia Reduced pitch and possibility of reduced loudness Difficult producing higher pitch notes Voice quality is worse with its use	In infant - mainly on pre-school ages, more in boys In adolescence – mainly at 10 years old, more in girls It could disappear after puberty Could develop muscle tension dysphonia
Recurrent Respiratory Papillomatosis (Most common cause of dysphonia associated to a benign neoplasia)	Epithelial over-growing (epithelial hiperplasia) in any part of the superior respiratory tract, mainly in the vocal folds Incomplete glottal closure – irregular configuration After some surgical interventions there could be scars and fibrosis of the vocal folds	Congenital, although it could appear on the first 10 years of life Chronic cough	Voice breaks Reduced mucosal wave Severe roughness and harshness Aphonia Higher pitch, when associated to rigidity Strain	Lesions with aggressive growing, persistent and recurrent Negative impact in breathing is usual Variable evolution of lesions and voice quality Etiology in mother-fetus transmission of the Human Papilloma Virus In pediatric age incidence is equal between gender

Classification (Lesion or Disorder)	Organic and Functional Disorders	Causes/Associated Behaviors	Aerodynamic and acoustic characteristics	Observations
Laryngomalacia	Tonus disorder of the laryngeal skeleton and/or intrinsic laryngeal muscles Paradox movements associated to breathing	Congenital	Neonatal stridor because of flaccid epiglottis and aryepiglottic folds Roughness Reduced pitch and loudness is possible	Could evolve spontaneously, reversible in the first month of life
Vocal fold paralysis	Disorder of the movement and/or tonus of the vocal fold, unilateral or bilateral Incomplete glottal closure – triangular gap, in all extension	Congenital or acquired (namely associated to laryngeal trauma)	Roughness and Breathiness, depending on the position of the paralysis, uni or bilateral Form normal voice to aphonia	Unilateral disorder is 4 to 5 times more frequent than the bilateral
Polyps	Benign mass lesion of the lamina propria, usually unilateral, in the middle of the vocal folds Could be sessile or pediculate	Continuous vocal traumatic behaviors or one, very intense, vocal abuse Dehydration Allergies Dry environments Pharyngo-Esophageal Reflux Medication (anti-inflammatory and hormonal treatments)	Roughness and breathiness Diplophonia (in the pediculate polyps, because of the vibratory asymmetry) Phono-asthenia Difficult producing higher pitch notes Voice quality is worse with its use Reduced vocal extension and tessitura Pitch and loudness changes depend on the lesion characteristics	In adolescence – mainly after 10 years old, more in girls Voice changes gradually Dysphonia severity depends on the size of the mass lesion, rigidity of the vocal fold and the grade of the affection of the lamina propria Could develop muscle tension dysphonia

Appendix II. (Continued)

Classification (Lesion or Disorder)	Organic and Functional Disorders	Causes/Associated Behaviors	Aerodynamic and acoustic characteristics	Observations
Allergies and Infections of the Superior Respiratory Tract	Mucosal disorder because of lack of histamine Laryngeal edema and/or of the vocal folds	Contact with polluted environments or with allergenic factors Dehydration Dry environments Pharyngo-Esophageal Reflux	Vocal disorder dependent on the mucosal inflammation Hiponasality (resonance disorder) Disorder of the mucosal wave Globus sensation Cough Aphonia	
Puberphonia or Mutational Dysphonia	Detailed description along the text			

References

Angelillo, N., Di Costanzo, B., Angelillo, M., Costa, G., Barillari, M. R., & Barillari, U. (2008). Epidemiological study on vocal disorders in paediatric age. *J. Prev. Med. Hyg.*, 49(1), 1-5.

Azevedo, R. (2010). Disfonia na Infância. In F. Fernandes, B. Mendes & A. Navas (Eds.), *Tratado de Fonoaudiologia*. São Paulo: Roca.

Behlau, M., Dragone, M. L., Ferreira, A., & Pela, S. (1997). Higiene vocal infantil - Informações básicas. São Paulo: Lovise.

Bhattarai, S., Sunil Kumar Shah. (2010). Psychosocial impact on puberphonic and effectiveness of voice therapy: A case report. *Journal of College of Medical Sciences-Nepal*, 6(1), 57-62.

Boseley, M. E., Cunningham, M. J., Volk, M. S., & Hartnick, C. J. (2006). Validation of the Pediatric Voice-Related Quality-of-Life survey. *Arch; Otolaryngol; Head Neck Surg;*, 132(7), 717-720.

Carding, P., Roulstone, S., Northstone, K., & Alspacstudyteam. (2006). The Prevalence of Childhood Dysphonia: A Cross-Sectional Study. *Journal of Voice,* 20(4), 623-630.

Connor, N., Cohen, S., Theis, S., Thibeault, S., Heatley, D., & Bless, D. (2008). Attitudes of Children With Dysphonia. *Journal of Voice*, 22(2), 197-209.

Cotes, C. (1997). O Mago das Vozes: Lovise.

De Bodt, M. S., Ketelslagers, K., Peeters, T., Wuyts, F. L., Mertens, F., Pattyn, J., et al. (2007). Evolution of Vocal Fold Nodules from Childhood to Adolescence. *Journal of Voice*, 21(2), 151-156.

Dejonckere, P.H.; Bradley, P.; Clemente, P. et al. (2001) A basic protocol for functional assessment of voice pathology, especially for investigating the efficacy of (phonosurgical) treatments and evaluating new assessment techniques. *Eur. Arch. Otorhynolaryngol.*, 258, 77-82.

Fuchs, M., Meuret, S., Thiel, S., Täschner, R., Dietz, A., & Gelbrich, G. (2009). Influence of Singing Activity, Age, and Sex on Voice Performance Parameters, on Subjects' Perception and Use of Their Voice in Childhood and Adolescence. *Journal of Voice*, 23(2), 182-189.

Gasparini, G., Behlau, M., & Azevedo, R. (2006). Era uma voz: TT THOT.

Graham, J. M., Scadding, G. K., & Bull, P. D. (Eds.). (2007). Pediatric ENT. Springer Science & Business Media.

Hartnick, C.J. (2002). Validation of a pediatric voice quality-of-life instrument: the pediatric voice outcome survey. *Arch. Otolaryngol. Head Neck Surg.*, 128, 919-922.

Marsal, C. A., & Vila, M. E. I. (2005). Disfonía infantil: diagnóstico y tratamiento: Ars Médica.

Martins, S. (n/d). Disfonia Infantil - Terapia: Revinter.

McAllister, A., Sederholm, E., Sundberg, J., & Gramming, P. (1994). Relations between voice range profiles and physiological and perceptual voice characteristics in ten-year-old children. *J. Voice*, 8(3), 230-239.

McNeil, M. R. (1997). *Clinical Management of Sensorimotor Speech Disorders*: Thieme.

Melo, A., Caeiro, M., Lavra, T. (2006). *A nossa Voz*. Lisboa: Hospital D. Estefânia.

Mitchell, R. B., & Pereira, K. D. (Eds.). (2009). Pediatric otolaryngology for the clinician. Humana.

Muniz, F., & Ono, W. (2010). Rita, Nao Grita! : Melhoramentos.

Roy, N., Holt, K. I., Redmond, S., & Muntz, H. (2007). Behavioral Characteristics of Children With Vocal Fold Nodules. *Journal of Voice,* 21(2), 157-168.

Schindler, A., Capaccio, P., Maruzzi, P., Ginocchio, D., Bottero, A., & Ottaviani, F. (2007). Preliminary considerations on the application of the Voice Handicap Index to paediatric dysphonia. *Acta Otorhinolaryngol.* Ital., 27(1).

Schindler, A., Capaccio, P., Maruzzi, P., Ginocchio, D., Bottero, A., & Ottaviani, F. (2007). Preliminary considerations on the application of the Voice Handicap Index to paediatric dysphonia. *Acta Otorhinolaryngol.* Ital., 27(1).

Schindler, A., Capaccio, P., Maruzzi, P., Ginocchio, D., Bottero, A., & Ottaviani, F. (2007). Preliminary considerations on the application of the Voice Handicap Index to paediatric dysphonia. *Acta Otorhinolaryngol.* Ital., 27(1).

Sederholm, E. (1996a). Hoarseness in Ten-Year-Old Children: Perceptual Characteristics, Prevalence and Etiology. Karolinska Institute, Huddinge University Hospital.

Sederholm, E. (1996b). Medical and socio-emotional factors related to chronic and acute hoarseness in ten-year-old children. *Manuscript submitted to publication.*

Sederholm, E. (1996c). Perceptual Evaluation of Connected Speech and Sustained Vowels in Children's Voice. *Manuscript submitted to publication.*

Sederholm, E., McAllister, A., Dalkvist, J., & Sundberg, J. (1995). Aetiologic factors associated with hoarseness in ten-year-old children. *Folia Phoniatr Logop,* 47(5), 262-278.

Seikel, J. A., King, D. W., & Drumright, D. G. (2010). *Anatomy & Phisiology fo Speech, Language,* and Hearing. New York: Delmar.

Simões, S. (2011). Especificidades do Canto no Ensiono Básico. Universidade de Aveiro, Aveiro.

Verdolini, K., Rosen, C. A., Rosen, C. A., & Branski, R. C. (Eds.). (2014). Classification manual for voice disorders-I. Psychology Press.

Verduyckt, I., Morsomme, D., Remacle, M. (2012). Validation and Standardization of the Pediatric Voice Symptom Questionnaire: A Double-Form Questionnaire for Dysphonic Children and Their Parents. *Journal of Voice*, 1-11.

Zur, K.B., Cotton, S., Kelchner, L., Baker, S., Weinsrich, B., Lee, L. (2007). Pediatric Voice Handicap Index (pVHI): a new tool for evaluating pediatric dysphonia. *Int. J. Pediatr Otorhinolaryngol.*, 71, 77-82.

In: Voice Disorders
Editor: Derrick Welch

ISBN: 978-1-63484-413-0

Chapter 4

STATE OF VOICE QUALITY IN PEDAGOGUES AT PRIMARY SCHOOLS

Kristýna Vojkovská[1,2], Mgr, Eva Mrázková[1,2,3,4], MUDr, PhD, and Petra Sachová[2,5], Mgr

[1]Department of Epidemiology and Public Health, Faculty of Medicine, University of Ostrava, Ostrava, Czech Republic
[2]Center for Hearing and Balance Disorders, Czech Republic
[3]Department of Otorhinolaryngology, Hospital and Polyclinic Havirov, Havirov, Karviná, Czech Republic
[4]Occupational Health and Preventive Medicine, University Hospital Ostrava, Ostrava, Czech Republic
[5]Faculty of Medicine and Dentistry, Palacký University, Olomouc, Czech Republic

ABSTRACT

Introduction: A cultivated vocal performance is one of the preconditions of succeeding in many professions. It is mainly used and hence strained by voice professionals for whom it is a work tool. An important group representing voice professionals is composed of pedagogues.

The objective of the thesis was a voice analysis of primary school pedagogues in the Czech region of Ostrava.

Methodology: A two-phase study was executed at Ostrava primary schools involving a computer voice analysis performed by means of the lingWAVES computer modular system for voice analysis and therapy. Participation in both phases of the study was based on voluntariness. In the first phase of the study 63 primary schools were approached. 34 primary schools from various city boroughs joined the project between September and November 2012, giving 495 respondents in total. 484 persons underwent an acoustic computer analysis of the voice, which is 98 per cent of respondents. Within the scope of the study's second phase the data collection took place in the second half of June 2013 with 2 primary schools from Poruba joining the project. The lower number in comparison with the first phase is caused by the pedagogues' commitments at the end of the school term, and by part of schools refusing to participate due to specifically abridged school terms. Altogether 19 respondents of the female sex were examined. The final comparison and results of the study included the same pedagogues as in the first and second phase of the study. The data was evaluated using statistical methods.

Results: By means of acoustic assessment of the speaking voice the following was judged – phonation time, intensity range, speaking profile and the vospector DSI (Dysphonia Severity Index). The difference in the results of phonation time between the two phases was insignificant. As regards intensity range and the speaking profile slope, a decrease in the quality of good voices was observed in the second phase of measuring. It is clear from the vospector DSI comparison that there is a difference between the first and second phase of the study in the number of pedagogues in groups 1 (constant dysphonia), 2 (moderate dysphonia), and 3 (slight to medium dysphonia).

Conclusion: The thesis considered the voice quality state by means of focusing on voice professionals, particularly primary school pedagogues. The most significant deterioration in voice quality was recorded in the vospector DSI parameter, where the number of pedagogues in the groups of constant, moderate and medium to slight dysphonia increased.

The results of the study confirm both a decline in voice dynamics and voice deterioration at the end of the school term.

The project was funded through the grant SMO 0211/2012/KZ: "Epidemiological study of the frequency of voice disorders in pedagogues and a proposal for its prevention" of the University of Ostrava and the Statutory City of Ostrava. The thesis should motivate voice professionals to take preventive measures and thus lower the number of injuries of the vocal apparatus.

INTRODUCTION

A cultivated speech and vocal performance is one of the preconditions of succeeding in many professions. Approximately one third of the employed population use their voice daily as a main work tool. We call them voice professionals, and their voice is to them the main means of work. Yet most people realise the importance of voice only when they start to have problems with it. In spite of the valuable scientific and technical progress, many aspects of modern everyday life remain to be extremely difficult to people with speech or voice disorder. An important group representing voice professionals is composed of pedagogues. The objective of the thesis was a voice analysis of primary school pedagogues in Ostrava by means of a standardised computer-operated measuring system.

The project was funded through the grant SMO 0211/2012/KZ: “Epidemiological study of the frequency of voice disorders in pedagogues and a proposal for its prevention” of the University of Ostrava and the Statutory City of Ostrava. Thanks to the project the participating pedagogues could verify their current voice possibilities. The thesis should motivate voice professionals to take preventive measures and thus lower the number of injuries of the vocal apparatus.

METHODOLOGY

The study focused on pedagogues or voice professionals at Ostrava primary schools. In the Czech Republic these belong to primary education.

The Czech Republic educational system is based on the School Act No. 561/2004 Coll. that provides for preschool, primary, high school, colleges and other education, and defines the process of gradual acquisition of qualification at individual stages of the schooling system. The main structure of the system divides education into three areas: primary (primary/elementary), secondary (grammar/high school), and tertiary (other).

Primary education is provided via a network of primary schools for children between 6 and 15 years of age. This nine-year school attendance is mandatory in the Czech Republic. This can be preceded by preschool education which is organised by nursery schools for children between the age of 3 and 6.

Primary education is followed by secondary education which usually lasts three or four years, although one-year or two-year courses do exist. Secondary education is provided by high schools which are categorised according to the method of graduation into high school education, high school education with vocational certificate, and high school education with maturita exam.

Tertiary education offers the possibility for maturita exam holders to improve their qualifications in various specialisations, by means of studying either at universities or colleges.

A teacher, or pedagogue, is one of the basic officials within the educational process who plans, organises, realises, and evaluates. In most European countries only a person with pedagogical education can become a teacher, and it is the same in the Czech Republic. One part of the whole body of pedagogical activities is language performance. The voice output of a teacher is strenuous and so places the profession among voice professional. By the term *voice professionals* we therefore understand people who need perfect voice function in order to practice their job. A voice professional is therefore a person whose profession is directly dependent on vocal communication. As regards voice quality demands, voice professionals are divided into four groups, which slightly vary according to different authors.

According to the Union of European Phoniatricians four groups of voice professionals are recognised from the viewpoint of voice quality:

1) singers – both soloists and chorus singers (maximum voice quality demand)
2) actors, professional spokespersons, teachers
3) judges, doctors, politicians, managers, the clergy
4) sellers, news vendors

According to Koufman of the Voice Institute of New York, voice professionals, in terms of voice quality level, are classified as follows:

1st level – elite professional artists (singers, actors)

2nd level – semi-professional elite voice artists (students of acting and singing)

3rd level – voice professionals (teachers, the clergy, managers, telephone operator)

4th level – voice semi-professionals (chorus singers, pedagogy students)

The classification of voice professionals does not take into account the intensity or length of needed voice performance, or the link between voice requirement and financial income. As far as speaking voice is concerned, voice professionals lay stress on strength and resilience of voice to load. In our study we focused on teachers – i.e., the first group according to Veld's classification, and the third level according to Koufman's classification – for whom high voice quality is a necessity [1, 2, 3].

According to the recommendation of the Union of European Phoniatricians, pedagogues fall within the second most demanding group of voice professionals in relation to voice quality requirements. A two-phase study was executed at Ostrava primary schools involving a computer voice analysis performed by means of the Voice Diagnostic Centre (VDC) Lingwaves computer modular system for voice analysis and therapy, in this case focusing on the speaking profile. Participation in both phases of the study was based on voluntariness and the approval of all primary school headmasters.

Within the scope of the study's first phase 63 primary schools in Ostrava were approached. 34 primary schools from various city boroughs joined the project between September and November 2012, giving 495 respondents in total. 484 persons underwent an acoustic computer analysis of the voice, which is 98% of respondents. Within the scope of the study's second phase the data collection took place in the second half of June 2013 with 2 primary schools from Poruba joining the project. The lower number in comparison with the first phase is caused by the teachers' commitments at the end of the school term, and by part of schools refusing to participate due to either specifically abridged school terms or scheduled construction works. Altogether 19 female respondents were examined. The final comparison and results of the study included the same pedagogues as in the first and second phase of the study.

Within the first phase of the study a questionnaire survey was conducted among the pedagogues. This had the form of an interview, when a communicator (competent examiner) put questions to a respondent (examined voice professional). The voice professional questionnaire was functionally composed so that it was as comprehensible as possible and not very long. It included a series of questions concerning personal, professional and family anamnesis, and consisted of 20 items in total. Collected personal data was handled in accordance with Act No. 177/2001 Coll., on the Protection of Personal Data and on Amendment to Some Acts in the wording of later legal regulations [4].

Voice and speech computer analysis, or phonetographic voice diagnostic centre, uses high quality software which enables voice recording. The Voice Diagnostic System (VDC) Lingwaves serves for a combined analysis of human voice using voice range profiles or phonetograms. Phonetogram represents a two-dimensional voice range analysis and can be used for voice quality assessment. VDC Lingwaves includes a sound pressure level meter that ensures higher accuracy of intensity measurement (IEC 651 type 2, suitable for laboratory and scientific tasks), so the intensity is read directly from the meter signal and digitally transferred for software processing. Therefore, no intensity calibration is required. For the purpose of pitch calculations an Electret condenser microphone was used, built into a sound level meter (SPL meter). The measuring is typically conducted at a 30 cm distance from the mouth. The phonetogram meets the requirements of the Union of European Phoniatricians for standardised phonetography [5, 6].

By means of acoustic speaking voice assessment the following parameters were considered – phonation time, intensity range, speaking profile and the vospector DSI (Dysphonia Severity Index). All required operations were recorded by the system and then evaluated. The measuring was always conducted in the quietest room of the school.

The speaking profile slope (SPS) is created by measuring soft, normal, loud, and shouting voice. In this way a client's average voice range is defined. The results are imaged as a curve showing how fast the pitch grows with increasing volume. Its slope informs us about voice quality. Steep increase of the curve represented by number value (i.e. curve slope ≥1) is typical for good voices [6]. The client was always asked slowly to count from 21 to 40 at first in normal, then soft and finally loud voice. The client was to avoid whispering in the soft voice and shouting in the loud voice. In the last phase the client was asked to shout, loud and long, the sentence "Hey, what are you doing there!" The shouting was to be as loud as possible, as if the client wanted to attract the attention of a friend walking on the other side of a busy street. It was important to bear in mind that the shouting voice was supposed to exceed 90dB. The calculations were shown as enclosed areas and crosses, where every cross was assigned a letter: "S" for soft voice, "N" for normal/calm, "L" for loud and "▲" for shouting voice (Figure 1).

The *Dysphonia Severity Index*, designed by Marc S. De Bodt and Floris L. Wyuts form the University of Antwerp, was measured as an objective and quantitative voice quality correlate. It is a parameter that was created as a result of attempts at an objectification of voice disorder assessments by one number.

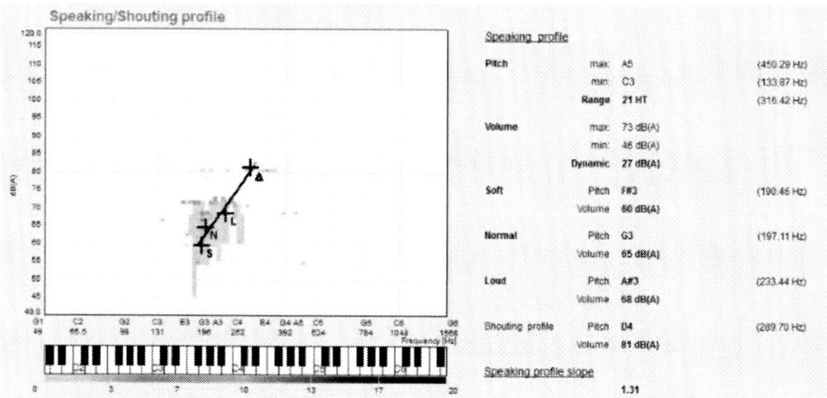

Figure 1. Speaking profile slope (SPS).

It combines several voice measurings into one individual measuring and it is construed as a weighted combination of four voice characteristics: maximum phonation time (MPT, s), highest frequency (F0-Hogh, Hz), lowest intensity (I-Low, dB), and jitter (%), Figure 2.

It is construed as:

DSI = 0.13 x MPT + 0.0053 x F0-High – 0.26 x I-Low – 1.13 x Jitter (%) + 12.4.

The mentioned group of 4 parameters was selected from a group of 45 parameters on the basis of a multivariate statistical analysis so, that their weighted linear correlation expressed a perception assessment of the overall voice disorder as well as possible. By means of the DSI index it is possible to classify voices into six classes of voice damage (Table 1) and it may be used for documenting changes in voice quality on a one-dimensional scale from 15 to – 5. The more negative a client's index value is, the more dysphonic his voice is considered to be. And vice versa – the higher the index value, the better the voice quality. The influence of gender is included indirectly in the calculation of DSI, therefore it is not necessary to use a separate index for men and women [7, 8].

A respondent was asked to produce a vowel sound (for instance "a") in a calm tone and hold it for at least 3-4 seconds. The highest frequency (F0-High, Hz) and the lowest intensity (I-Low, dB/A) from the SPS measuring were automatically available for an overall calculation of DSI.

Table 1. Voice classification according to Dysphonia Severity Index [6]

GROUP	DSI RANGE	DESCRIPTION
0	<-2,0	Severe persistent aphonia: patient unable to produce voice
1	-1,9 až +0,3	Constant dysphonia: sporadic periods of phonation, aphonic periods may occur
2	+0,4 až 2,2	Moderate dysphonia: patient able to produce voice, but frequent periods of dysphonia occur
3	+2,3 až +3,3	Slight to medium dysphonia: less frequent periods of disturbed phonation or light persistent dysphonia
4	+3,4 až +4,3	Slight dysphonia: sporadic moments of dysphonia in short periods
5	>4,4	No dysphonia

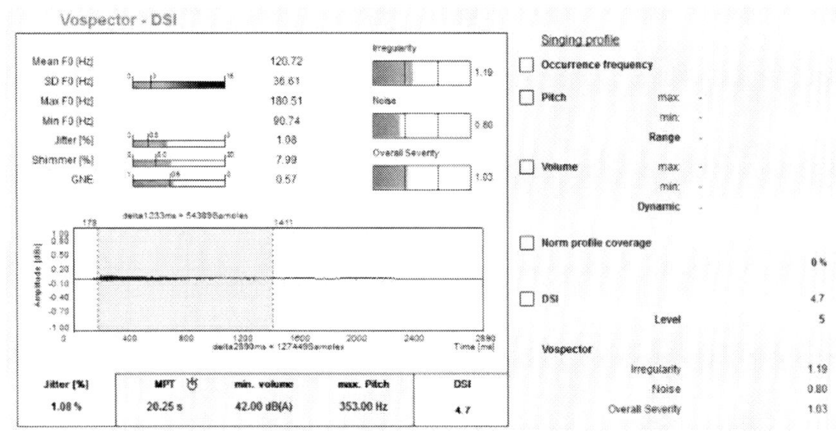

Figure 2. Dysphonia Severity Index (DSI).

Phonation time, one of the functional features of the voice, is the time in seconds for which a particular person, having taken one breath, is able to sustain an intermittently sung (phonated) tone. With the common breath-in, the average phonation time in an adult lasts 15-20 seconds, in singers it reaches 40-60 seconds [9, 10]. The respondents were asked to produce a long calm tone while we measured the time that elapsed since the beginning until the end of phonation.

Intensity or dynamic voice range is the difference between maximal and minimal measured acoustic pressure levels during a given voice task. The softest phonations are mostly possible at lower pitch, while the loudest at high or middle pitch. This depends on the level of trainedness and the voice pathology type. If we work on the usual values for a healthy, untrained voice, on average it ranges between 20 to 28 dB in men, and between 18 to 28 dB in women. Values about 8 dB are considered pathological. The average dynamic voice range in 25 dB [9, 11, 12]. We learnt these values during the measuring of DSI.

The data collected during the conducted measurings was transferred into Microsoft Office Excel in the form of a database. The statistical evaluation too was done in Microsoft Office Excel.

In the case of quantitative data the basic characteristics were calculated (arithmetic mean, standard deviation, minimal and maximal value) and methods of regression and correlation analysis used. Further statistical tests: two-sample F-test for equality of two variances, two sample t-test for equality of expected value with equal or unequal variances, one-way ANOVA variance analysis, test for independence. The significance level was set at 5%.

In the case of qualitative data frequency analysis was conducted (absolute and relative values). Contingency tables were used and Pearson's contingency coefficient calculated for the evaluation of qualitative data dependence. Statistical tests: test for independence, goodness-of-fit-tests (Pearson's chi-squared test, Kolmogorov-Smirnov test). The significance level was again set at 5%. The results are transferred into charts and accompanied with statistical evaluation.

RESULTS

Parameters collected by the acoustic assessment of speaking voice in all 19 pedagogues that participated in both phases of the study were processed and statistically evaluated.

Characteristics of population: the maximum and minimum age limit was individually restricted by the transaction of business. Population age range was between 26 and 64 years, the average age was 50 years (SD ± 2.19). Some respondents transacted their business during old age pension. All respondents were of the female sex. At the same time, all pedagogue were educated at university. Maximum practice time in respondents reached 38 years, while minimum just 1 year. Average business transaction time amounted to 24 years

(SD ± 2.2). The number of pupils in class ranged from 7 to 30, on average there were 16 pupils per class (SD ± 1.9). The lowest and highest number of a pedagogue's lessons in one day depended on the pedagogue's number of hours of working time and timetable. Within minimum number of hours the results ranged between 2 and 4 lessons per day (SD ± 0.18). Within maximum lessons per day the lowest value reached 2 lessons per day, while the highest was 7 lessons per day (SD ± 0.26). On average there were 4.3 lessons per day (SD ± 0.21). From the voice professionals population 26% of persons (N = 5) had not undergone any phoniatric examination so far, and none of the remaining 74% of voice professionals (N = 14) that had experienced a phoniatric examination in the past, went for a preventive voice examination.

The smoking habit among voice professionals was distributed in the following way. Non-smokers were prevalent in the voice professionals population, i.e., 84% (N = 16), 11% of voice professionals (N = 2) were ex-smokers, and only 5% of pedagogues (N = 1) were smokers. Due to the low number of smokers we supposed that a smoking habit would not show on the voice condition, which was confirmed by statistical evaluation. To the question whether the respondents viewed their own voice rather as higher (soprano) or lower (alt), the pedagogues answered as follows: 16% of pedagogues (N = 3) placed their voices among the higher, while 84% (N = 16) among the lower.

By means of subjective speaking voice quality assessment the pedagogues were sorted in the following way: 5% of voice professionals (N = 1) were fully satisfied with their voice quality, 11% (N = 2) were rather satisfied, 79% (N = 15) were rather dissatisfied and 5% of population, i.e. 1 pedagogue, wasn't satisfied at all. According to the evaluation of their vocal resonation, 79% of voice professionals (N = 15) described their voice as full and 21% of population (N = 4) as hoarse. The other two options, asthenic voice and aphonia were not selected by any of the pedagogues.

Power-based voice production by means of increased outer muscle tension, pain and discomfort during phonation were felt by 16% of voice professionals population (N = 3), the remaining part of population (84%, N = 16) did not suffer from these problems.

According to voice hygiene self-assessment the respondents were divided as follows: 5% of population (N = 1) had excellent knowledge in this field, 21% (N = 4) claimed to have very good knowledge, 37% of pedagogues (N = 7) saw their knowledge as good. 32% of population (N = 6) had small knowledge of voice hygiene and the knowledge of 5% (N = 1) was insufficient.

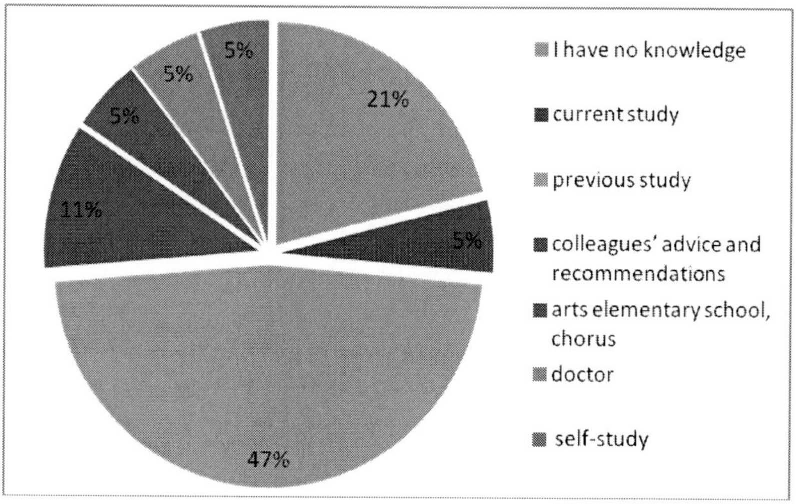

Chart 1. Source of voice hygiene knowledge for voice professionals.

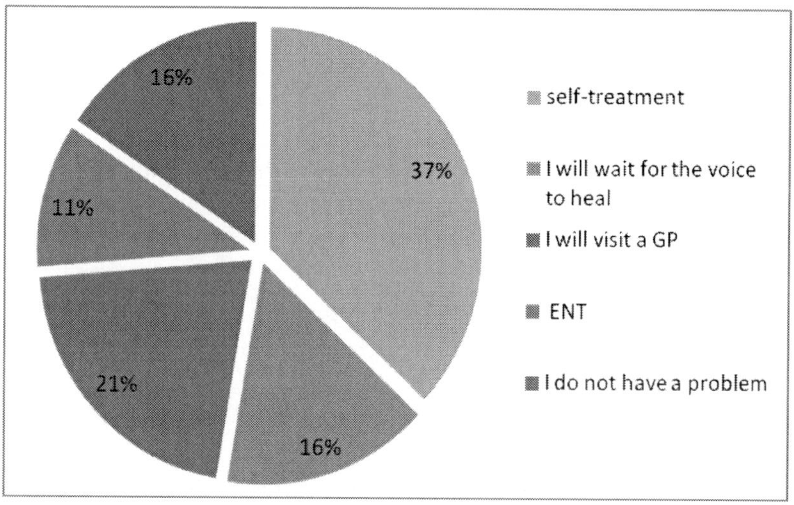

Chart 2. Ways of solving voice problems in voice professionals.

Previous study of the subject was the most common source of voice hygiene knowledge for 47% of pedagogues (N = 9), followed by a chance of studying now, i.e., while gaining qualification as part of pedagogical practice (21%, N = 4), then colleagues' advice and recommendations (11%, N = 2). Specific figures are given in Chart 1. 37% of pedagogues (N = 7) chose the 'self-treatment' option as a solution to their voice problems, followed by 'I will visit a GP' (21%, N = 4), and 'I will wait for the voice to heal' in third (16%, N = 3). The same part of population (16%, N = 3) stated they did not have any problem, Chart 2.

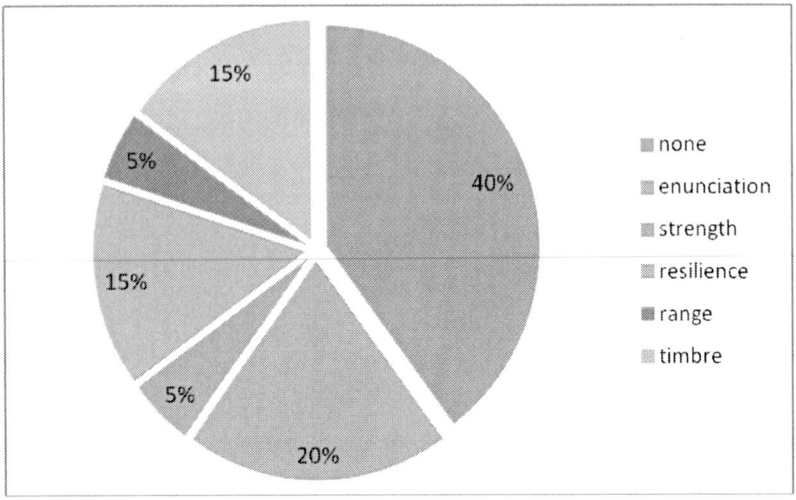

Chart 3. Perceived need of voice change.

To the question what the perceived need of voice change was the most common answer was 'none' (40%, N = 8), further followed enunciation (20%, N = 4) and the equally resilience and timbre (15%, N=3), Chart 3.

During self-assessment of speech activities 21% of pedagogues (N = 4) described themselves as quiet and taciturn persons, further 68% (N = 13) as average speakers and the remaining 11% of population (N = 2) described themselves as talkative persons.

Maximum phonation time was measured as below average in 8 pedagogues (42%) during the first phase of the study. 6 respondents (32%) reached average values, and the remaining 5 respondents (26%) acquired above average values. The lowest measured value of phonation time was measured at 9.25 seconds, while the highest value was 30.3 seconds. During the second phase of the study 5 pedagogues (26%) reached average phonation time. 8 persons (42%) showed below average values, and 6 persons (32%) reached above average values. The lowest phonation time value was measured at 5.35 seconds, and the highest measured value was 38.25 seconds. Diaphragmatic breathing was evident in persons that showed above average phonation time values. By contrast, below average results corresponded with thoracic breathing.

The results from both phases of measuring were not significant in any way, Chart 4. The phonation time median was 17 seconds in the first phase (SD ± 5.41), 18.19 seconds in the second phase (SD ± 8.27), Chart 5, where blue values represent the so called outliers.

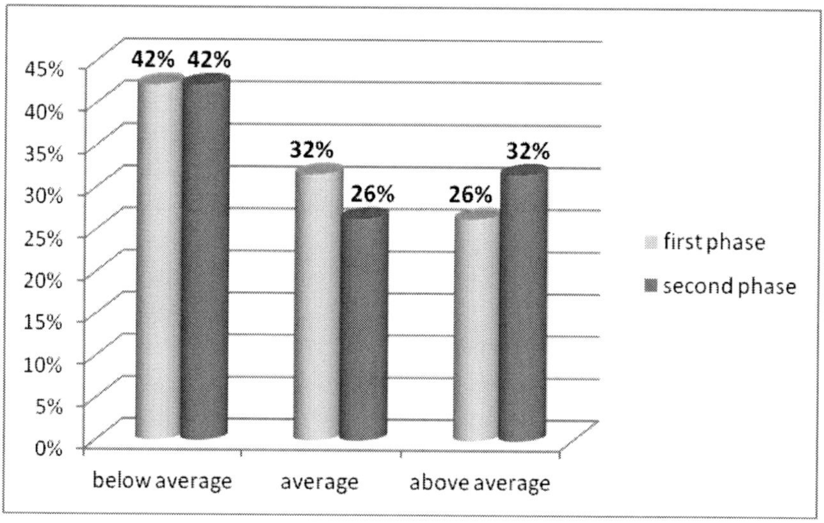

Chart 4. Phonation time of pedagogues in the first and second phase of study.

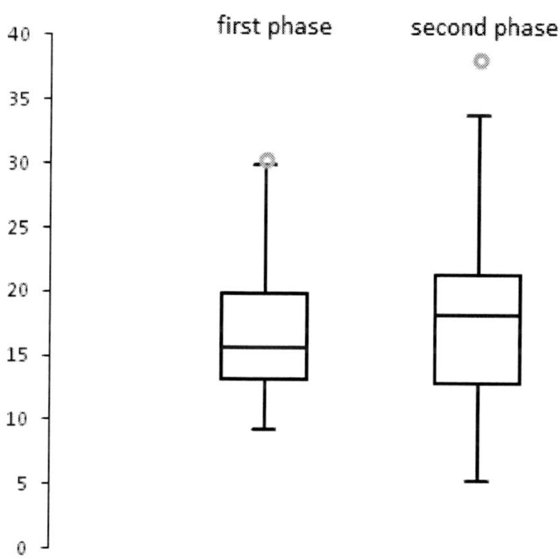

Chart 5. Phonation time values of pedagogues in the first and second phase of study.

For statistical processing the following null hypothesis H0 was set: There is no difference in the phonation time values in the first and second phase of measuring.

At a 5% significance level it was shown, by means of both a two-sided (p-value 0.6183) and a one-sided (p-value 0.3091) paired two-sample mean-comparison t-test, that we do not reject the H0 hypothesis. There is no statistically significant difference in phonation time values in the first and second phase of the study.

Another parameter gained from the measuring is *intensity or dynamic range*. During the study's first phase, majority of persons (13 pedagogues, 68%) reached average values. 1 respondent (5%) reached below average, but not pathological values, and 5 pedagogues showed above average intensity range (26%). The lowest intensity value recorded was 42 dB, while the highest value was 102 dB. In the second phase of the study 9 pedagogues (47%) reached average values, 4 pedagogues (21%) reached below average but not pathological values, and 6 pedagogues (32%) showed above average intensity range. The lowest intensity recorded was 42 dB, while the highest was 89 dB. Here we recorded an increase in persons with below average intensity range in the second phase of the study, Chart 6. In the first phase the average dynamic range value is 24.74 dB (SD ± 4.86), in the second phase of the study it is 25.37 (SD ± 8.43), Chart 7.

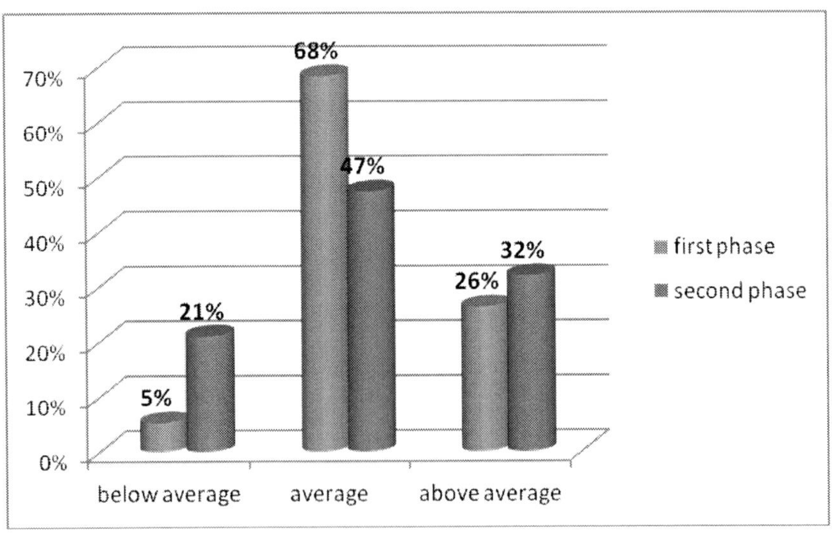

Chart 6. Dynamic range of pedagogues during the first and second phase.

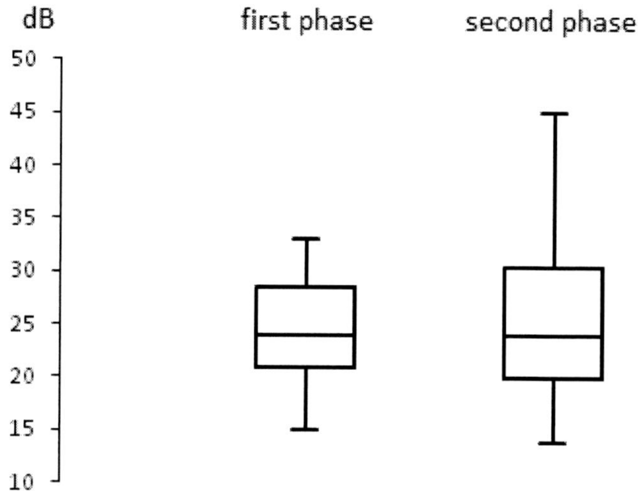

Chart 7. Average values of Dynamic values of pedagogues during the first and second phase.

For statistical processing the following null hypothesis H0 was set: There is no difference in average dynamic range values (in dB) in the first and second phase of study. At a 5% significance level it was shown, by means of both a two-sided (p-value 0.8051) and a one-sided (p-value 0.4026) paired two-sample mean-comparison t-test, that we do not reject the H0 hypothesis.

There is no statistically significant difference in values of the average dynamic range in the first and second phase of the study.

In the *speaking profile slope* parameter 3 persons (16%) measured a value lower than 1 and 16 respondents (84%) showed a value higher than 1 in the first phase of the study. In the second phase of the study 11 persons (58%) corresponded with good voice quality (value > 1). 8 persons (42%) measured values below 1. In the second phase we can again see a decrease in good voice quality, Chart 8. The average value for speaking profile slope in the first phase of the study is 1.69 (SD ± 1.75), while in the second phase of the study 0.67 (SD ± 2.31), Chart 9, where the blue points represent the outliers and red crosses represent distant extreme values.

For statistical processing the following null hypothesis H0 was set: There is no difference in speaking profile slope values in the first and second phase of study.

At a 5% significance level it was shown, by means of a two-sided paired two-sample mean-comparison t-test, that we do not reject the H0 hypothesis.

There is no statistically significant difference in speaking profile values in the first and second phase of the study (p-value 0.0908).

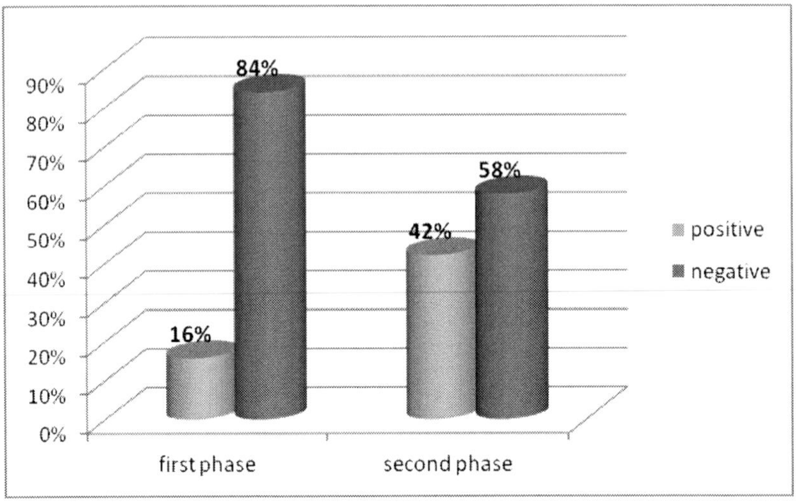

Chart 8. Speaking profile slope of pedagogues in the first and second phase of the study.

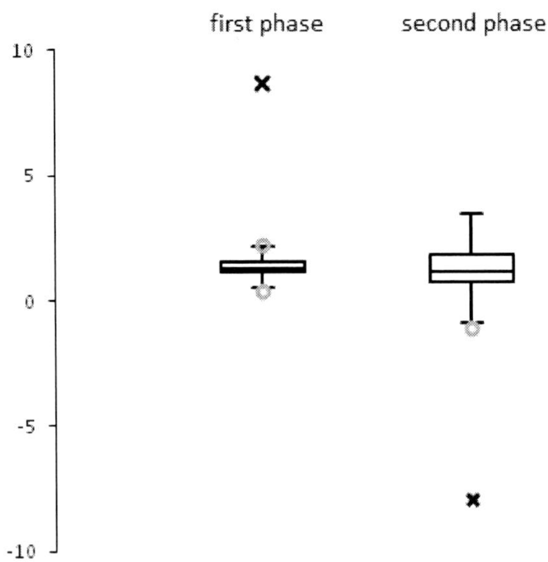

Chart 9. Pedagogues' speaking profile slope values in the first and second phase of the study.

The result of a one-sided paired two-sample t-test comparing the speaking profile slope means is that the average of values measured in the 1st phase of study is higher than the average of values measured in the 2nd phase of study (p-value 0.0454).

As regards *dysphonia severity index,* the resulting values reflected individual groups in the first phase of the study as follows: 5 – no dysphonia in 12 pedagogues (67%); 4 slight dysphonia in 5 pedagogues (28%); 3 – slight to medium dysphonia in 1 pedagogue (6%); 2 – moderate dysphonia, 1 – constant dysphonia, and 0 – severe persistent aphonia in 0 pedagogues (0%). In one person a complete combination of four voice characteristics was unnecessary for index calculation.

In relation to measuring in the second phase of the study the resulting values reflected individual groups in the following way: 5 – no dysphonia in 2 pedagogues (12%); 4 slight dysphonia in 2 pedagogues (12%); 3 – slight to medium dysphonia in 5 pedagogue (29%); 2 – moderate dysphonia in 4 pedagogues (24%), 1 – constant dysphonia in 4 pedagogues (24%), and 0 – severe persistent aphonia in 0 pedagogues (0%). It was not possible to obtain a final value in 2 persons due to an incomplete combination of four voice characteristics necessary for index calculation.

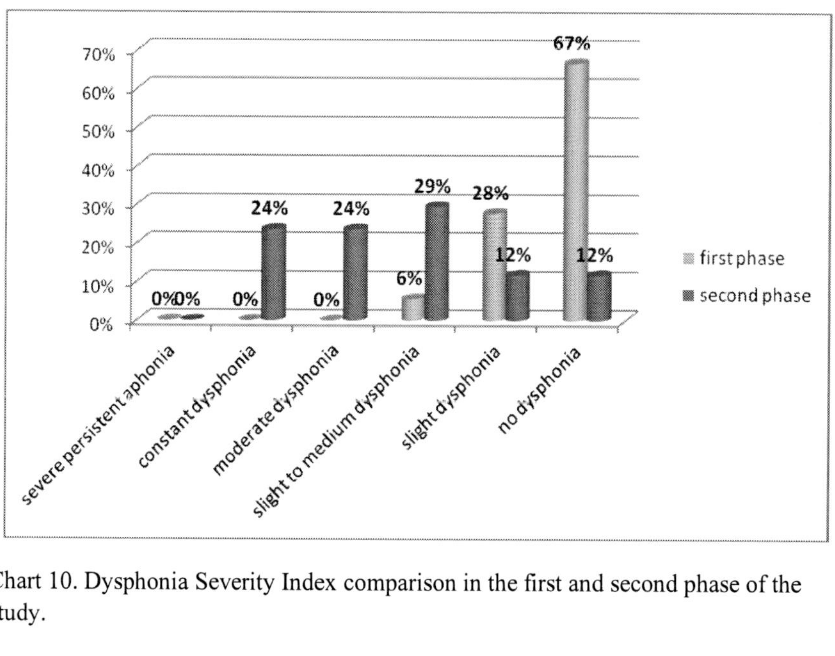

Chart 10. Dysphonia Severity Index comparison in the first and second phase of the study.

Chart 10 clearly shows there is a difference between the first and second phase of the study in that the number of pedagogues in groups 1 (constant dysphonia), 2 (moderate dysphonia), and 3 (slight to medium dysphonia) increased in the second phase of measuring. The Dysphonia Severity Index mean in the first phase of the study is 5.081 (SD ± 1.32), in the second phase it is 2.063 (SD ± 2.15), Chart 11. For statistical processing the following null hypothesis H0 was set: There is no difference in Dysphonia Severity Index values in the first and second phase of study.

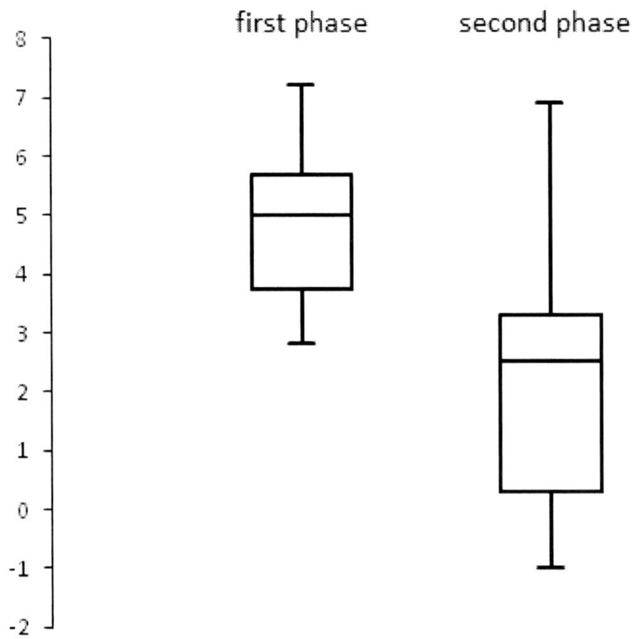

Chart 11. Dysphonia Severity Index values in the first and the second phase of the study.

At a 5% significance level it was shown, by means of both a two-sided (p-value 8.38E-05) and a one-sided (p-value 4.19E-05) paired two-sample mean-comparison t-test, that we reject the H0 hypothesis. There is a statistically significant difference in Dysphonia Severity Index values in the first and second phase of the study. The result of a one-sided paired two-sample mean-comparison t-test is that the average of Dysphonia Severity Index values measured in the first phase of the study is higher than the average of Dysphonia Severity Index values measured in the second phase of the study.

Acoustic voice analysis by means of the Vospector module offers a quick way to obtain data on various phonetographic values on the basis of which an overall condition or overall voice damage are generated. In our study we focused on irregularity or roughness, noise (breathiness) or voicelessness and overall damage or hoarseness. The results were divided into three categories – moderate, medium, and severe problems in the particular area. In the first phase of our study irregularity was spread among our 19 selected respondents in the following way: 11 pedagogues (58%) had moderate problems, 8 pedagogues (42%) suffered from medium problems and severe problems were present in none. Irregularity measuring corresponds with the perceived voice roughness. Noise measuring gives a voice breathiness overview. In our population 16 pedagogues (84%) showed low noise energy and the other 3 respondents (16%) high noise energy. In our population overall damage was recorded as moderate in 14 pedagogues (74%) and as severe in 5 pedagogues (26%). Overall results of damage measuring correlate with perceived hoarseness. Jitter, a periodic oscillation of basic frequency, was moderate in all 19 pedagogues (100%). In the second phase of the study 18 pedagogues underwent the Vospector module acoustic voice analysis. Irregularity was spread among the respondents as follows: 11 pedagogues had moderate problems (58%), 7 pedagogues medium (37%), and severe none. Irregularity measurements correlate with the perceived roughness. Noise measuring gives a voice breathiness overview. In our population all 18 pedagogues (95%) showed low noise energy.

By means of statistical evaluation in the first and second phase of irregularity, noise, and jitter study no statistically significant difference was confirmed.

Overall damage was shown in our population as moderate in 15 pedagogues (79%) and as severe in 3 pedagogues (16%). Overall results of damage measuring correlate with perceived hoarseness. Periodic oscillation of basic frequency – jitter – was moderate in 16 pedagogues (84%) and severe in 2 pedagogues (11%).

Here we did not record any significant difference between the first and the second phase of measuring. The average value of overall damage in the first phase of the study was 0.932 (SD ± 0.20), in the second phase it was 0.857 (SD ± 0.13), Chart 12.

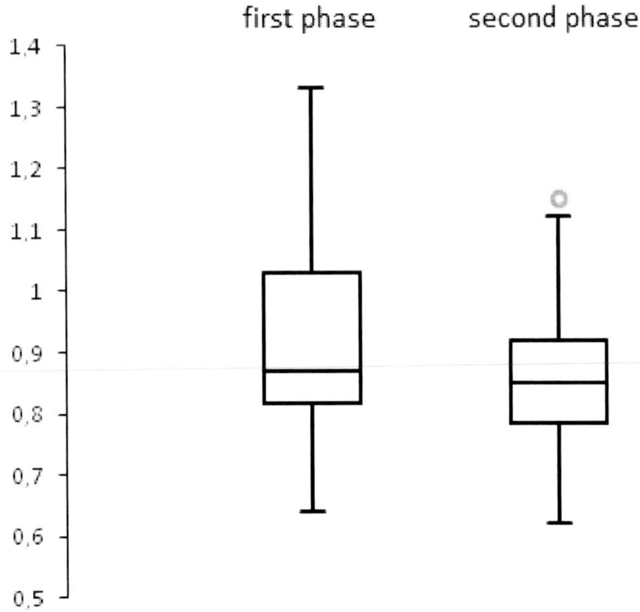

Chart 12. Overall damage from the first and second phase of the study.

For statistical processing the following null hypothesis H0 was set: There is no difference in overall damage values in the first and second phase of study.

At a 5% significance level it was shown, by means of both a two-sided (p-value 0.2000) and a one-sided (p-value 0.1000) paired two-sample mean-comparison t-test, that we do not reject the H0 hypothesis. There is no statistically significant difference in values of overall damage in the first and second phase of the study.

Discussion

In spite of growing technological progress, the voice has taken over an important role not only in business activities during the past decades. Due to this fact voice disorders not only affect the careers of many voice professionals, but also lower the profit of their employers. That is why recently the topic of voice as a work tool, vocal care, and last but not least its therapy, has attracted more attention not only from a medical, but also a social and an economical point of view [13]. In our modern lifestyle more than 20% of economically active population use voice as the main tool in their professional activities. For instance, data from the United Kingdom shows that more than 5 million workers are affected by voice disorders at an annual cost of £200 mil. [14].

The voice of pedagogues has been the subject of many studies all over the world, as teachers are an attractive statistical population in the field of professional voice disorders. Notwithstanding all the research on the subject of voice problems in teachers, the occurrence of voice disorders within this group is still rather an unknown variable and accounts of their appearance cover a wide range. Considerably more works on the evaluation of professional singing voice than of speaking voice were published. Yet the results of studies agree on the prevalence of voice disorders in teachers in comparison with other professions. For example, in her study, Cecilia Pemberton mentions three- to five-times higher likelihood of voice disorder occurrence in teachers than in common population. Another author, Niebudek-Bogusz, mentions in her research five-times higher prevalence of voice disorders in teachers than in the control group [15-23]. Our population was represented by primary school teacher.

In Poland, professional voice disorders are the most frequent category of professional disorders – they consist 20% of all cases [18]. In the Czech Republic, 52 professional voice disorders were reported as occupational disease between the years 1996 and 2014. A more detailed analysis showed that the highest number of voice disorders in the given period was among pedagogues, with women being the most afflicted. Women prevail in the pedagogical profession according to other researches, too [24, 25]. In our study the population of voice professionals consist only of women. It is evident that the female sex dominates the pedagogical profession.

The objective DSI voice evaluation that was used in our study is used abroad as an orientation tool signalling changes in voice quality. The DSI method has been used so far mainly for phoniatric patients at various rehabilitation programmes, but experience indicates it could also be used for people whose profession entails voice load, for instance teachers [26]. In objective Dysphonia Severity Index voice evaluation by means of a voice diagnostic centre it is not necessary to compare differences between the sexes, since the effect of the sex is indirectly included in the DSI calculation, according to Wuyts. However, it was mentioned in many other researches that women suffered from voice problems more often than their male counterparts [7, 27-30]. Hence was confirmed the higher accumulation of professional disorders in women substantiated, according to many authors, by their more frequent work with younger children [28, 31, 32]. Our results can neither confirm nor refute this fact due to the zero occurrences of men in our population.

Particularly nursery and primary school teachers are considered to be representative of a profession with high voice load, and according to Laukkanen, Pekkarinen et al. they form 16% of all voice professionals [30, 33]. One of the factors is the use of voice at its full strength intelligibly for many hours daily. According to authors Bermúdez de Alvear, Sala, or Viljanen, teachers spend up to 90% of their working time in oral explanation. As a matter of fact, they use their voice at high intensity, in loud classrooms and for a long time without proper breaks [34, 35]. Overloading of the vocal apparatus was confirmed by other studies [36-39]. Daily voice load of voice professionals in our population depended on their transaction of business, on average 4.3 lessons per day (SD ± 0.21). The lowest voice load per day the pedagogues stated was most commonly 2-4 lessons, while the highest voice load stated was 2-7 lesson per day. In the work of authors Pešlová and Brhel it is claimed that professional voice disease was diagnosed and reported on average after 21.2 years of pedagogical practice [40]. The average length of practice in our population was 24 years (SD ± 2.2).

Based on DSI, in the fisrt phase of the study 33% of pedagogues suffered from various forms of dysphonia, from light, through moderate, to constant dysphonias, but in the second phase of the study it was already 88% of population. The increase in worse values of the dysphonia severity index was statistically proved. This fact is a predisposition for vocal apparatus pathology or even for originating a professional voice disorder, according to Sliwinska-Kowalska [41].

Maximum phonation time is an important variable for overall voice quality evaluation, according to Wuyts et al. The obtained values divided our population into three groups with the designation 'below average', 'average', and 'above average maximum phonation time'. Both in the first and the second phase of the study 42% of population reached below average maximum phonation time. The number of pedagogues with average maximum phonation time slightly dropped in the second phase of the study, from 32% to 26%, while the number of pedagogues with above average maximum phonation time rose from 26% to 32%. The statistical difference between the first and the second phase of the study was insignificant. Maximum phonation time is relative to the correct use of breath and to the vocal folds size [16]. Diaphragmatic breathing was evident in persons that showed above average phonation time values, and by contrast, below average results corresponded with thoracic breathing. A fact verified by Lejska was confirmed, that the better the breathing activity, the longer the phonation and vice versa [16]. A correct breathing activity belongs to vocal education knowledge.

One third of pedagogues assessed their level of voice hygiene as small, and one voice professional even described it as insufficient. The range of voice hygiene knowledge in the studied sample of teachers does not reach a level that could be expected in expert pedagogues. In a questionnaire survey the pedagogues stated they would like to improve or change the articulation, resilience, or timbre of their voice.

Dr Inez Kozelské states that teachers do not seek professional phoniatric consultation during frequently accumulated voice disorders [42]. Among the voice professionals in our population 37% of respondents marked 'self-treatment', which was the most common solution to voice disorders, followed by 'I will visit a GP' in 21% of pedagogues, and the same number of pedagogues stated they had no problem that would require any treatment. Only 11% of respondents chose an ENT doctor, and a specialised phoniatric care was chosen by none of the voice professional.

Among teachers, voice disorders are considered to be occupational hazard in a matter-of-course way, yet the exact etiology of voice disorder origination is still under investigation and the subject of many studies. Individual researches emphasise many influencing factors. Up to date it has not been made clear which factors play the biggest role in the development of voice problems and consequent disorders not only among teachers. More and more people use their voice as one of the main work tools in their profession. It is important to start with voice hygiene at a time when the voice is well. Studies prove that teachers who had some voice training complain less about the symptoms of voice problems, and more hours of vocal courses or education is connected with a lower rate of reporting voice problems [15, 18, 43-47]. According to Niebudek-Bogusz voice training is a decisive method of voice therapy and its knowledge may sufficiently compensate for professional voice load [45]. Programmes should mainly concentrate on preventive measures and education in the field of voice hygiene. Training attitudes should be individual with the length, content and intensity adapted to a particular client and his/her problems. The integration of vocal courses into a lifelong learning programme could perhaps lead to the maximization of voice health, especially of voice professionals.

Conclusion

The voice of pedagogues is a rather current topic in the field of professional voice disorders. Particularly a teacher's profession is responsible and demanding, as the teacher is entrusted with very valuable articles – children, and thus their and our future. By definition the teacher should meet professional requirements. Especially in the case of pedagogues voice care and education should be as pragmatic as possible. The results of many studies indicate that teaching is a high-risk profession leading to voice disorders and that this health issue may be connected to an inability to practise the profession and consequent economical impact.

The goal of this work was an assessment of voice loading and voice quality evaluation in voice professionals, Ostrava primary school pedagogues.

It was determined that teachers perceive speaking voice disorders. According to an objective measuring by means of VDC and Dysphonia Severity Index, 33% pedagogues during the first and 88% during the second phase of the study suffered from various forms of dysphonia, from slight and moderate to severe dysphonia. It was the biggest deterioration in all the studied parameters. By means of DSI evaluation it was statistically confirmed that voice quality deteriorated towards the end of the term. In the other parameters the differences in the second phase of the study were not statistically significant.

A big part of pedagogues in the third largest city of the Czech Republic – Ostrava – do not know how to work with their voice and how to care for it. Pedagogues themselves describe their voice hygiene knowledge as low, or even insufficient. Voice professionals in our population want to improve or change the articulation, resilience, and timbre of their voice. Teachers should be generally informed about the symptoms of potential voice problems, so that they may undergo professional medical examination and appropriate treatment in time.

The results of the study show that the voice condition of teachers is not at a level their profession requires. The current problem, then, is not only the search for methods, procedures, principles, and measures that would lead to healthy voice sustenance and voice condition recovery, but that would also motivate to timely and responsible voice care.

References

[1] Dršata, Jakub. Foniatrie - hlas. 1. vyd. Havlíčkův Brod: Tobiáš, 2011, 321 s. *Medicína hlavy a krku*, ISBN 978-80-7311-116-8.

[2] Koufman, J. A.; Isaacson, G. The spectrum of vocal dysfunction. *Otolaryngologic Clinics of North America*, 1991, 24.5: 985-988.

[3] Veldová, Zuzana. Možnosti léčby hlasových profesionálů v ambulantní praxi. Interní medicína pro praxi. 2005, č. 11, s. 496-498. Dostupný z WWW: <http://www.internimedicina.cz/artkey/int-200511-0007.php >.

[4] Zákon č. 177/2001 Sb. o ochraně osobních údajů a o změně některých zákonů, dostupné na URL: <http://www.mvcr.cz/sbirka/2001/sb067-01.pdf>.

[5] Sulter, Arend M., Harm K. Schutte, Donald G. Miller, Christine Sheard, Louis Heylen, Benoite Millet, Kristiane Van Lierde, Jan Raes a Paul H. Van de Heyning. Differences in phonetogram features between male and female subjects with and without vocal training: A Challenge for Occupational Safety and Health Arrangement. *Journal of Voice,* 1995, 9(4): 363-377. DOI: 10.1016/S0892-1997(05)80198-5. ISSN 08921997.

[6] WEVOSYS: Speech and Voice Assessment Tools [online]. *Forchheim Germany,* 2014 [cit. 2015-07-20]. Dostupné z: http://wevosys.com/ index.html.

[7] Hakkesteegt, M. M. (2009, October 7). Evaluation of Voice Disorders: Dysphonia Severity Index and Voice Handicap Index. Erasmus University Rotterdam. ISBN 978-90-9024566-9. Retrieved from http://hdl.handle.net/1765/16932.

[8] Wuyts, Floris L., Marc S. De Bodt, Geert Molenberghs, Marc Remacle, Louis Heylen, Benoite Millet, Kristiane Van Lierde, Jan Raes a Paul H. Van de Heyning. The Dysphonia Severity Index: A Challenge for Occupational Safety and Health Arrangement. *Journal of Speech Language and Hearing Research,* 2000, 43(3): 796-. DOI: 10.1044/ jslhr.4303.796. ISSN 1092-4388.

[9] Kejklíčková, Ilona. Logopedie v ošetřovatelské praxi. Vyd. 1. Praha: Grada, 2011, 128 s. Sestra (Grada). ISBN 978-80-247-2835-3.

[10] Lejska, Mojmír. Poruchy verbální komunikace a foniatrie. Brno: Paido, 2003. ISBN 80-7315-038-7.

[11] Frič, M.: Porovnání parametrů hlasových polí u hlasových profesionálů a začínajících studentů herectví, Proceeding of the 4th International Symposium Material – Acoustics – Place 2008, Technical University in Zvolen, 2008, s. 47-52.

[12] Kučera, Martin, Marek Frič a Martin Halíř. Praktický kurz hlasové rehabilitace a reedukace. Opočno: M. Kučera, 2010, 57 l. ISBN 978-80-254-6592-9.

[13] Šram, František, Jan G. Švec a Jitka Vydrová. Včasná diagnostika poruch hlasu včetně rakoviny hlasivek. Zdraví E15: Příloha: Lékařské listy [online]. 2010, (3). Dostupné z: http://zdravi.e15.cz/clanek/priloha-lekarske-listy/vcasna-diagnostika-poruch-hlasu-vcetne-rakoviny-hlasivek-449628.

[14] Carding, Paul. Occupational voice disorders: Is there a firm case for industrial injuries disablement benefit?. *Logopedics Phoniatrics Vocology,* 2007, 32.1: 47-48.

[15] Boltežar, Lučka; Šereg Bahar, Maja. Voice Disorders in Occupations with Vocal Load in Slovenia/Glasovne Težave V Poklicih Z Glasovno Obremenitvijo V Sloveniji. *Slovenian Journal of Public Health*, 2014, 53.4: 304-310.

[16] Lejska, Mojmír, Eva Bártková, Radan Havlík, Pavla Weberová a Jana Frostová. DSI – Dysphonia Severity Index. In: Audio-Fon Centr. [online]. Brno, 2010 [cit. 2015-06-27]. Dostupné z: http:// www.audiofon.cz/odborna-innost-pracovit/pednaky/38-dsi-dysphonia-severity-index-.html.

[17] Morton, Valerie; Watson, David R. The teaching voice: problems and perceptions. *Logopedics Phoniatrics Vocology*, 1998, 23.3: 133-139.

[18] Niebudek-Bogusz, Ewa; Śliwińska-Kowalska, Mariola. An overview of occupational voice disorders in Poland. *International journal of occupational medicine and environmental health,* 2013, 26.5: 659-669.

[19] Pekkarinen, Eeva, Lea Himberg, Jaana Pentti, Christine Sheard, Louis Heylen, Benoite Millet, Kristiane Van Lierde, Jan Raes a Paul H. Van De Heyning. Prevalence of vocal symptoms among teachers compared with nurses: A questionnaire study. *Logopedics Phoniatrics Vocology,* 1992, 17(2): 113-117. DOI: 10.3109/14015439209098721. ISSN 1401-5439.

[20] Pemberton, Cecilia. Voice Injury in Teachers: Voice Care Prevention Programmes To Minimise Occupational Risk [online]. 2010. Dostupné z: http://www.voicecareaustralia.com.au/Voice%20Injury%20in%20 Teachers.pdf.

[21] Titze, Ingo R.; Lemke, Julie; Montequin, Doug. Populations in the US workforce who rely on voice as a primary tool of trade: a preliminary report. *Journal of Voice*, 1997, 11.3: 254-259.

[22] Verdolini, Katherine; Ramig, Lorraine O. Review: occupational risks for voice problems. *Logopedics Phonatrics Vocology*, 2001, 26.1: 37-46.

[23] Smith, Elaine, Steven D. Gray, Heather Dove, Lester Kirchner, Heidi Heras, Benoite Millet, Kristiane Van Lierde, Jan Raes a Paul H. Van De Heyning. Frequency and effects of teachers' voice problems: A questionnaire study. *Journal of Voice*, 1997, 11(1): 81-87. DOI: 10.1016/S0892-1997(97)80027-6. ISSN 08921997.

[24] Gkalpakioti, Petra. Profesionální poškození zdraví u žen. Praha, 2009. Dostupné také z: https://is.cuni.cz/webapps/zzp/detail/49979/?lang=en Diplomová práce. Univerzita Karlova v Praze. Vedoucí práce Doc. MUDr. Monika Kneidlová, CSc.

[25] Státní Zdravotní Ústav. Nemoci z povolání v České republice [online]. Dostupné z: http://www.szu.cz/publikace/data/nemoci-z-povolani-a-ohrozeni-nemoci-z-povolani-v-ceske-republice.

[26] Frostová, Jana. Zkušenosti s měřením kvality hlasu pomocí DSI - Dysphonia Severity Index. In: AUDIO - Fon Centr. [online]. Brno, 2010. Dostupné z: http://www.audiofon.cz/odborna-innost-pracovit/pednaky.html?format=html&limitstart=30.

[27] Angelillo, Italo Francesco, et al. Prevalence of occupational voice disorders in teachers. *Journal of preventive medicine and hygiene*, 2015, 50.1.

[28] Preciado-López, Julián, Carmen Pérez-Fernández, Miguel Calzada-Uriondo, Pilar Preciado-Ruiz, Heidi Heras, Benoite Millet, Kristiane Van Lierde, Jan Raes a Paul H. Van De Heyning. Epidemiological Study of Voice Disorders Among Teaching Professionals of La Rioja, Spain: A questionnaire study. *Journal of Voice*, 2008, 22(4): 489-508. DOI: 10.1016/j.jvoice.2006.11.008. ISSN 08921997.

[29] Roy, Nelson. Functional dysphonia. *Current Opinion in Otolaryngology and Head and Neck Surgery,* 2003, 11.3: 144-148.

[30] Vilkman, Erkki, Jennifer Oates, Kenneth M. Greenwood, Lester Kirchner, Heidi Heras, Benoite Millet, Kristiane Van Lierde, Jan Raes a Paul H. Van De Heyning. Occupational Safety and Health Aspects of Voice and Speech Professions: A questionnaire study. *Folia Phoniatrica et Logopaedica*, 2004, 56(4): 220-253. DOI: 10.1159/000078344. ISSN 1421-9972.

[31] Roy, Nelson, Ray M. Merrill, Susan Thibeault, Rahul A. Parsa, Steven D. Gray a Elaine M. Smith. Prevalence of Voice Disorders in Teachers and the General Population. *Journal of Speech Language and Hearing*

Research, 2004, 47(2): 281-. DOI: 10.1044/1092-4388(2004/023). ISSN 1092-4388.

[32] Vilkman, Erkki. Voice Problems at Work: A Challenge for Occupational Safety and Health Arrangement. *Folia Phoniatrica et Logopaedica*, 2000, 52(1-3): 120-125. DOI: 10.1159/000021519. ISSN 1421-9972.

[33] Laukkanen A.-M. On speaking voice exercises. A study on the acoustic and physiological effects of speaking voice exercises applying manipulation of the acoustic-aerodynamical state of the supraglottic space and artificially modified auditory feedback [doctoral dissertation]. Tampere:University of Tampere, 1995.

[34] Bermúdez de Alvear RM: Perfil de uso vocal en el profesorado de los colegios públicos de Málaga (in Spanish), thesis, Malaga, 2003.

[35] Sala, E. a V. Viljanen. Improvement of acoustic conditions for speech communication in classrooms. *Applied Acoustics*, 1995, 45(1): 81-91. DOI: 10.1016/0003-682X(94)00035-T. ISSN 0003682x.

[36] Bermúdez De Alvear, Rosa M.; Barón, Francisco Javier; Martínez-Arquero, Antonio Ginés. School teachers' vocal use, risk factors, and voice disorder prevalence: guidelines to detect teachers with current voice problems. *Folia phoniatrica et logopaedica*, 2011, 63.4: 209-215. ISSN 1421-9972.

[37] Rantala, Leena, Erkki Vilkman a Risto Bloigu. Voice Changes During Work. *Journal of Voice*, 2002, 16(3): 344-355. DOI: 10.1016/S0892-1997(02)00106-6. ISSN 08921997.

[38] Roy, Nelson, et al. Voice disorders in the general population: prevalence, risk factors, and occupational impact. *The Laryngoscope,* 2005, 115.11: 1988-1995.

[39] Södersten, Maria, Svante Granqvist, Britta Hammarberg a Annika Szabo. Vocal Behavior and Vocal Loading Factors for Preschool Teachers at Work Studied with Binaural DAT Recordings. *Journal of Voice,* 2002, 16(3): 356-371. DOI: 10.1016/S0892-1997(02)00107-8. ISSN 08921997.

[40] Pešlová, Marie, Brhel, Petr. Profesionální poruchy hlasu . Pracovní lékařství [online]. 2002, č. 1, s. 21-23. Dostupný z WWW: http://www.prolekare.cz/pracovni-lekarstvi-clanek/profesionalni-poruchy-hlasu-29435?confirm_rules.

[41] Sliwinska-Kowalska, M., E. Niebudek-Bogusz, M. Fiszer, T. Los-Spychalska, P. Kotylo, B. Sznurowska-Przygocka a M. Modrzewska. The Prevalence and Risk Factors for Occupational Voice Disorders in

Teachers. *Folia Phoniatrica et Logopaedica*, 2006, 58(2): 85-101. DOI: 10.1159/000089610. ISSN 1421-9972.

[42] Kozelská, Inez. Hlasová výchova v učitelské přípravě: (jako dovednostní součást profesionalizace učitelů 21. století). Vyd. 1. V Ostravě: Ostravská univerzita, Pedagogická fakulta, 2004. ISBN 978-807-0423-592.

[43] Frostová, Jana, et al. Changes of the quality of voice in nursery school teachers measured by the DSI and VHI methods: Evaluation on completion of a training programme. *School and Health*, 2011, 21: 151-161.

[44] Leão, Sylvia H. S., et al. Voice problems in New Zealand teachers: a national survey. *Journal of Voice*, 2015.

[45] Niebudek-Bogusz, E., et al. The effectiveness of voice therapy for teachers with dysphonia. *Folia Phoniatrica et Logopaedica*, 2008, 60.3: 134-141.

[46] Niebudek-Bogusz, Ewa, et al. Acoustic analysis with vocal loading test in occupational voice disorders: outcomes before and after voice therapy. *International journal of occupational medicine and environmental health*, 2008, 21.4: 301-308.

[47] Smolander, Sini; Huttunen, Kerttu. Voice problems experienced by Finnish comprehensive school teachers and realization of occupational health care. *Logopedics Phoniatrics Vocology*, 2006, 31.4: 166-171.

BIBLIOGRAPHY

A primer on communication and communicative disorders LCCN: 2010050452 Personal name: Schwartz, Howard D., 1950- author. Main title: A primer on communication and communicative disorders / Howard D. Schwartz, Northern Illinois University. Published/Created: Boston: Pearson Education, Inc., [2012], ©2012. Description: xxi, 299 pages: illustrations; 24 cm. ISBN: 9780205496365 0205496369 LC classification: RC423 .S258 2012 Contents: Communication and communicative disorders -- Anatomy and physiology of speech, language, and voice production -- Speech sounds, articulation, and phonological disorders -- Language development in children -- Language disorders in children -- Communication in a multicultural society -- Neurological impairment: speech and language disorders in adults -- Voice disorders -- Swallowing disorders -- Fluency disorders -- Anatomy and physiology of hearing and hearing disorders -- Hearing testing and management of hearing disorders. Subjects: Communicative disorders. Speech therapy. Audiology. Communication Disorders. Communication. Notes: Includes bibliographical references (pages 283-289) and index. Series: The Allyn & Bacon Communication Sciences and Disorders Series.

Body and voice: somatic re-education LCCN: 2014005111 Personal name: Gilman, Marina, author. Main title: Body and voice: somatic re-education / Marina Gilman, MM, MA, CCC-SLP,; illustrations by Alex

Rowe; medical illustrations by Peggy Firth. Published/Produced: San Diego, CA: Plural Publishing, Inc., [2014] ©2014 Description: xiii, 252 pages: illustrations; 23 cm + 1 CD-ROM (4 3/4 in.) ISBN: 9781597565097 (alk. paper) 1597565091 (alk. paper) LC classification: RF510 .G55 2014 Contents: The somatic awareness: body and voice working as one -- Body and voice: somatic and physiologic connections -- The significance of the unremarkable -- Diversionary, parasitic, or other unnecessary preparatory movements -- Releasing for breathing -- Mobilizing the pelvis -- Improving stability. Subjects: Voice disorders. Voice Training. Exercise Movement Techniques--methods. Movement--physiology. Voice Disorders--therapy. Voice Quality--physiology. Notes: "Audio recordings of all the lessons presented in this book are included in the accompanying CD"--Page 4 of cover. Includes bibliographical references and index.

Choral pedagogy LCCN: 2013006760 Personal name: Smith, Brenda (Brenda Jo), author. Main title: Choral pedagogy / Brenda Smith, DMA, Robert T. Sataloff, MD, DMA, FACS. Edition: Third edition. Published/Produced: San Diego: Plural Publishing, [2013] Description: xiv, 322 pages: illustrations; 23 cm ISBN: 9781597565356 (alk. paper) 1597565350 (alk. paper) LC classification: MT875 .S63 2013 Related names: Sataloff, Robert Thayer, author. Contents: Amateur and professional choral singers -- The rehearsal process -- Anatomy and physiology of the voice -- Medical care of voice disorders / Robert T. Sataloff and Mary Hawkshaw -- Hearing loss in singers and other musicians / Robert T. Sataloff, Joseph Sataloff, and Caren J. Sokolow -- The aging voice / Margaret Baroody and Brenda Smith -- Performing arts medicine and the professional voice user -- Seating problems of vocalists / Richard Norris -- Historical overview of vocal pedagogy / Richard Miller -- Choral pedagogy and vocal health -- Voice disorders among choral music educators / Brenda Smith -- Singing in the 21st Century -- Choral singing and children -- The young singer / Vincent Oakes -- Voice building for choirs -- Choral singing -- Choral singing techniques -- Choral diction -- Rehearsal techniques -- The value of lifelong singing / Brenda Smith. Subjects: Choral singing--Instruction and study. Choral conducting. Voice--Care and hygiene. Voice Disorders--prevention & control. Singing--physiology. Vocal Cords--physiology. Voice--physiology. Voice Training. Notes: Includes bibliographical references (pages 287-291) and index.

Clinical management of children's voice disorders LCCN: 2009044501 Main title: Clinical management of children's voice disorders / [edited by] Christopher J. Hartnick and Mark E. Boseley. Published/Created: San Diego: Plural Pub., c2010. Description: x, 279 p.: col. ill.; 25 cm. ISBN: 9781597563543 (alk. paper) 1597563544 (alk. paper) LC classification: RF511.C45 C55 2010 Related names: Hartnick, Christopher J. Boseley, Mark E. Contents: Developmental, gross, and histologic anatomy of the larynx / Mark E. Boseley and Christopher J. Hartnick -- Pediatric laryngology: the office and operating room setup / Mark E. Boseley and Christopher J. Hartnick -- The pediatric speech pathologist and the hoarse child: evaluating the child with a voice disorder / Shirley Gherson and Barbara Wilson-Arboleda -- Voice quality of life instruments / Mark E. Boseley and Christopher J. Hartnick -- Laryngopharyngeal reflux and the voice / Stephen C. Hardy -- The role of the pediatric pulmonologist / Kenan E. Haver -- Laryngeal electromyography in pediatric patients / Al Hillel -- Pediatric laryngeal electromyography supplement / Andrew R. Scott and Christopher J. Hartnick -- Pediatric voice therapy: reviewing the data / Katherine Verdolini Abbott ... [et al.] -- Working with the pediatric singer: a holistic approach / Robert Edwin -- Benign lesions of the pediatric vocal folds: nodules, webs, and cysts / J. Scott McMurray -- Juvenile onset recurrent respiratory papillomatosis / Matthew T. Brigger -- Vocal fold immobility / Matthew T. Brigger and Christopher J. Hartnick -- Pediatric airway reconstruction and the voice / Karen B. Zur -- Functional and spasmodic dysphonias in children / Marshall E. Smith, Nelson Roy, and Cara Sauder -- Diagnosis and treatment of velopharyngeal insufficiency / Matthew T. Brigger, Jean E. Ashland, and Christopher J. Hartnick -- Paradoxical vocal fold motion / Venu Divi, Mary J. Hawkshaw, and Robert T. Sataloff -- Psychiatric and psychological interventions for pediatric voice disorders / Abigail L. Donovan and Bruce J. Masek. Subjects: Voice disorders in children. Voice Disorders. Child. Voice--physiology. Notes: Includes bibliographical references and index.

Clinical voice pathology: theory and management LCCN: 2009030698 Personal name: Stemple, Joseph C. Main title: Clinical voice pathology: theory and management / Joseph C. Stemple, Leslie E. Glaze, and Bernice Klaben. Edition: 4th ed. Published/Created: San Diego, CA: Plural Pub., c2010. Description: xv, 410 p., [12] p. of plates: ill. (some col.); 26 cm. ISBN: 9781597563482 (alk. paper) 159756348X (alk. paper) LC classification: RF510 .S74 2010 Related names: Glaze, Leslie E. Klaben, Bernice. Contents: Voice: a historical perspective -- Anatomy and physiology -- Some etiologic correlates -- Pathologies of the laryngeal mechanism -- The diagnostic voice evaluation -- Instrumental measurement of voice -- Survey of voice management -- The professional voice -- Rehabilitation of the laryngectomized patient. Subjects: Voice disorders. Voice Disorders. Notes: Includes bibliographical references and index.

Communication disorders in multicultural and international populations LCCN: 2011021819 Main title: Communication disorders in multicultural and international populations / [edited by] Dolores E. Battle; with 16 contributing authors. Edition: 4th ed. Published/Created: St. Louis, Mo.: Elsevier/Mosby, c2012. Description: ix, 326 p.: ill.; 29 cm. ISBN: 9780323066990 (alk. paper) 0323066992 (alk. paper) LC classification: RC423 .C6425 2012 Related names: Battle, Dolores E. Contents: Communication disorders in a multicultural and global society / Dolores E. Battle -- African American and other Blacks with communication disorders / Dolores E. Battle -- Communication disorders in Asian and Pacific American cultures / Li-Rong Lilly Cheng -- Communication disorders in the Middle East and Arab American populations / Freda Wilson -- Communication disorders in Native American and world wide indigenous cultures / Carol Westby, Ella Inglebret -- Hispanic and Latino cultures in the United States and Latin America / Hortencia Kayser -- Multilingual speech and language development and disorders / Helen Grech, Sharynne McLeod -- Neurogenic disorders of speech, language, cognition-communication, and swallowing / Constance Dean Qualls -- Cultural diversity and fluency disorders / Tommie L. Robinson Jr. -- International and intercultural aspects of voice and voice disorders / Marla Behlau, Thomas Murray -- Multicultural aspects of hearing loss / Zenobia Bagli -- Assessment of multicultural and international clients / Toya Wyatt -- Intervention for multicultural and international clients / Priscilla Nellum-Davis, Tachelle Banks -- Multicultural and international research: past, present, and future / Constance Dean Qualls. Subjects: Communicative disorders--United States. Transcultural medical care--United States. Multiculturalism--United States. Communication Disorders--ethnology. Cultural Diversity. Linguistics. Speech-Language Pathology--methods. Notes: Includes bibliographical references and index.

Communication sciences and disorders: an evidence-based approach LCCN: 2013444513 Personal name: Justice, Laura M., 1968-, author. Main title: Communication sciences and disorders: an evidence-based approach / Laura M. Justice, The Ohio State University, Erin E. Redle, Cincinnati Children's Hospital Medical Center, the University of Cincinnati. Edition: Third Edition. Published/Produced: Boston Pearson, [2014] ©2014 Description: xviii, 557 pages: illustrations; 26 cm. ISBN: 9780133123715 0133123715 LC classification: RC423 .J87 2014 Related names: Redle, Erin E., author. Review: "Introduces students to the field through clinicians, patients, and families. Rich with examples, the first part covers foundational concepts of development, anatomy, physiology, augmentative communication and complex communication. Following these foundations, the second part highlights inherited and acquired disorders affecting children and older adults. A new chapter features multicultural topics, while an expanded chapter delves into advancements in assessment and intervention. Strong themes of literacy weave throughout. Expanded cased keep student interest with evaluation and treatment sections." -- Back cover. Contents: Pt. I. Foundations of Communication Sciences and Disorders -- Ch. 1. Fundamentals of Communication Science and Disorders -- Ch. 2. An Overview of Communication Development -- Ch. 3. Anatomical and Physiological Bases of Communication and Communication Disorders -- Ch. 4. Augmentative and Alternative Communication -- Ch. 5. Communication Disorders in a Multicultural World -- Pt. II. Communication Disorders Across the Life Span -- Ch. 6. Communication Assessment and Intervention: Evidence-Based Practices Ch. 7. Language Disorders in Early and Later Childhood -- Ch. 8. Adult Language Disorders and Cognitive-Based Dysfunctions -- Ch. 9. Speech Sound Disorders in Children -- Ch. 10. Fluency Disorders -- Ch. 11. Voice Disorders -- Ch. 12. Motor Speech Disorders -- Ch. 13. Pediatric Hearing Loss -- Ch. 14. Hearing Loss in Adults -- Ch. 15. Feeding and Swallowing Disorders. Subjects: Communicative disorders. Speech disorders. Language disorders. Notes: Previously published as Communication sciences and disorders: a contemporary perspective, 2010. Includes bibliographical references and indexes.

Communication sciences and disorders: an introduction to the professions LCCN: 2011014074 Personal name: Williams, Dale F. Main title: Communication sciences and disorders: an introduction to the professions / Dale F. Williams. Published/Created: New York: Psychology Press, c2012. Description: xi, 436 p.: ill.; 24 cm. ISBN: 9780805861815 (hardback: alk. paper) 0805861815 (hardback: alk. paper) LC classification: RC428.5 .W55 2012 Summary: "I'll begin with the most general and work my way deductively to more specific terms. Communication--the processes by which information is exchanged (speaking, writing, semaphore, etc.). Disorder--a disturbance of structure, function, or both (Dirckx, 1997) (or, to state it differently: Something's wrong). Communication disorder--impairment in the ability to receive, process, represent, or transmit information (Nicolosi, Harryman, & Kresheck, 1989) (Something's wrong with communication. More specifically, something is wrong with speech, language, or hearing. By the way, the term communication disorders quite often applies to the field of study that encompasses speech-language pathology and audiology. I've been using communication sciences and disorders because 1) I strongly believe that the element of science is crucial to our understanding of communication and 2) that's the name of the department in which I'm employed. Language disorders--disorders affecting 1) the way you say (or write) your message and/or 2) your ability to understand the messages of others. Speech disorders--disorders affecting how one verbally produces language. These include impairments of articulation (sound pronunciation), fluency (most often stuttering), resonance (such as nasality--think Fran Drescher), or voice (e.g., hoarseness--Rod Stewart--or breathiness--Marilyn Monroe [Sorry youngsters;"--Provided by publisher. Subjects: Speech therapists--Practice. Communication disorders. Speech-Language Pathology. Communication Disorders. Communication. Hearing Disorders. Voice Disorders. Notes: Includes bibliographical references and indexes.

Diagnosis and evaluation in speech pathology LCCN: 2010054088 Personal name: Haynes, William O. Main title: Diagnosis and evaluation in speech pathology / William O. Haynes, Rebekah H. Pindzola. Edition: 8th ed. Published/Created: Upper Saddle River, N.J.: Pearson, c2012. Description: ix, 422 p.: ill.; 24 cm. ISBN: 9780137071326 (alk. paper) 0137071329 (alk. paper) LC classification: RC423 .H3826 2012 Related names: Pindzola, Rebekah H. (Rebekah Hand) Contents: Introduction to diagnosis and evaluation: philosophical issues and general guidelines -- Interviewing -- Psychometric considerations in diagnosis and evaluation -- Assessment of children with limited language -- Assessment of school-age and adolescent language disorders -- Assessment of speech sound disorders -- Disorders of fluency -- Assessment of aphasia and adult langauge disorders -- Motor speech disorders, dysphagia, and the oral exam -- Laryngeal and alaryngeal voice disorders -- Assessment of resonance imbalance -- Multicultural issues in assessment -- The diagnostic report. Subjects: Speech disorders--Diagnosis. Speech disorders--Case studies. Speech Disorders--diagnosis. Notes: Includes bibliographical references (p. 367-409) and index. Series: The Allyn & Bacon communication sciences and disorders series Allyn & Bacon communication sciences and disorders series.

Diagnosis and treatment of voice disorders LCCN: 2013049321 Main title: Diagnosis and treatment of voice disorders / [edited by] John S. Rubin, MD, FACS, FRCS, Robert T. Sataloff, MD, DMA, FACS, Gwen S. Korovin, MD, FACS. Edition: Fourth edition. Published/Produced: San Diego: Plural Publishing, Inc., [2014] ©2014 Description: xvii, 1019 pages: illustrations; 29 cm ISBN: 9781597565530 (alk. paper) 1597565539 (alk. paper) LC classification: RF510 .D53 2014 Related names: Rubin, John S. (John Stephen), editor of compilation. Sataloff, Robert Thayer, editor of compilation. Korovin, Gwen S., editor of compilation. Subjects: Voice disorders--Diagnosis. Voice disorders--Treatment. Laryngeal Diseases--diagnosis. Voice Disorders--diagnosis. Laryngeal Diseases--therapy. Larynx. Voice Disorders--therapy. Voice. Notes: Includes bibliographical references and index.

Exercises for voice therapy LCCN: 2013004663 Main title: Exercises for voice therapy / Alison Behrman, editor; John Haskell, editor. Edition: 2nd ed. Published/Created: San Diego, CA: Plural Pub., c2013. Description: xxi, 216 p.: ill.; 28 cm. + 1 sound disc (digital; 4 3/4 in.) ISBN: 9781597565301 (alk. paper) 159756530X (alk. paper) LC classification: RF510 .E94 2013 Related names: Behrman, Alison. Haskell, John, 1937- Contents: The practice of voice therapy -- Before and after -- Teaching speech breathing support -- Using a semi-occluded vocal tract -- Resonant voice -- Integrating voice production with body movement -- Articulatory freedom -- Teaching loud voice production -- Facilitating efficient vocal fold closure -- Pediatric voice therapy -- Special cases. Subjects: Voice disorders--Exercise therapy. Voice Disorders--therapy. Exercise Therapy--methods. Voice Training. Notes: Includes bibliographical references and index.

Geriatric otolaryngology LCCN: 2014044051 Uniform title: Geriatric otolaryngology (Sataloff) Main title: Geriatric otolaryngology / [edited by] Robert T. Sataloff, Michael M. Johns III, Karen M. Kost. Published/Produced: New York: Thieme, [2015] Description: p.; cm. ISBN: 9781626239777 (alk. paper) LC classification: RF47.A35 Related names: Sataloff, Robert Thayer, editor. Johns, Michael M., III, editor. Kost, Karen M., editor. Contents: The science of aging / Alessandro Bitto, Chad A. Lerner, and Christian Sell -- Geriatric otolaryngology: an overview / Karen M. Kost -- Understanding geriatric syndromes, the geriatric interdisciplinary team, and resources to optimize care for older patients / Sarah H. Kagan -- Evaluation of the outpatient geriatric patient / David Eibling -- Operative evaluation of the geriatric patient / Natalie Justicz and Jeanne Hatcher -- Age-related hearing loss / Kourosh Parham, Frank R. Lin, and Brian W. Blakley -- Regenerative therapies for sensorineural hearing loss: current research implications for future treatment / Cynthia L. Chow and Samuel P. Gubbels -- Hearing aids: considerations in the geriatric population / Amanda Kantor, Erica Miele, John Luckhurst, Mary Hawkshaw, and Robert T. Sataloff -- Cochlear implantation in the elderly / Daniel H. Coelho and Brian J. McKinnon -- Subjective idiopathic tinnitus in the geriatric population / Paul F. Shea and Brian J. McKinnon -- Dizziness, imbalance, and age-related vestibular loss in the geriatric population / Yuri Agrawal, Allan Rubin, and Stephen J. Wetmore -- Sinonasal disease in the elderly / David R. Edelstein -- Taste and smell in the elderly / Richard L. Doty and Hussam Tallab -- Inhalant allergies and asthma in the geriatric population / Karen H. Calhoun -- Voice disorders in the elderly / Robert T. Sataloff and Karen M. Kost -- Swallowing disorders in the elderly / Ozlem E. Tulunay-Ugur -- Sleep disturbance in the geriatric population / Christopher G. Larsen and M. Boyd Gillespie -- Facial plastic surgery in geriatric patients / J. Regan Thomas -- Oral cavity disorders in geriatric patients / Elliot Regenbogen and Denise A. Trochesset -- Advanced cutaneous malignancies in the elderly / Kelly Michele Malloy and Chaz L. Stucken -- Head and neck cancer in the elderly / Mihir R. Patel, Raymond L.

Chai, and Ara A. Chalian -- The role of neuropsychology in the evaluation and treatment of geriatric patients / Thomas Swirsky-Sacchetti and Caterina B. Mosti. Subjects: Otorhinolaryngologic Diseases. Aged.

Handbook of voice assessments LCCN: 2011009652 Main title: Handbook of voice assessments / [edited by] Estella Ma and Edwin Yiu. Published/Created: San Diego: Plural Pub., c2011. Description: xvi, 362 p.: ill.; 26 cm. ISBN: 9781597563642 (alk. paper) 1597563641 (alk. paper) LC classification: RF510 .H36 2011 Related names: Ma, Estella, 1975- Yiu, Edwin, 1958- Subjects: Voice disorders--Handbooks, manuals, etc. Voice Disorders--diagnosis--Handbooks. Notes: Includes bibliographical references and index.

International perspectives on voice disorders LCCN: 2012036460 Main title: International perspectives on voice disorders / edited by Edwin M-L. Yiu. Published/Produced: Bristol: Multilingual Matters, [2013] Description: xi, 203 pages: illustrations; 24 cm. ISBN: 9781847698735 (hbk: alk. paper) LC classification: RF510 .I58 2013 Related names: Yiu, Edwin, 1958- editor of compilation. Subjects: Voice disorders--Cross-cultural studies. Notes: Includes bibliographical references. Series: Communication disorders across languages.

INTRO: a guide to communication sciences and disorders LCCN: 2009036445 Personal name: Robb, Michael P. Main title: INTRO: a guide to communication sciences and disorders / Michael P. Robb. Published/Created: San Diego: Plural Pub., c2010. Description: xvi, 440 p.: ill. (some col.), col. maps; 27 cm. ISBN: 9781597563390 (alk. paper) 1597563390 (alk. paper) LC classification: RC423 .R57 2010 Portion of title: Guide to communication sciences and disorders Contents: Communication science -- Communication disorders and the professions -- Anatomic processes of speech and hearing -- Child language disorders -- Child phonological disorders -- Fluency disorders -- Cleft lip and palate -- Voice disorders -- Neurogenic communication disorders -- Dysphagia -- Genetics and syndromes -- Hearing disorders -- Auditory rehabilitation. Subjects:

Communicative disorders. Speech therapy. Audiology. Communication Disorders. Hearing Disorders. Notes: Includes bibliographical references and index.

INTRO: a guide to communication sciences and disorders LCCN: 2013033491 Personal name: Robb, Michael P., author. Main title: INTRO: a guide to communication sciences and disorders / Michael P. Robb, PhD. Edition: Second edition. Published/Produced: San Diego, CA: Plural Publishing Inc., [2014] ©2014 Description: xiv, 463 pages: illustrations (some color); 27 cm ISBN: 9781597565424 (alk. paper) 1597565423 (alk. paper) LC classification: RC423 .R57 2014 Variant title: Guide to communication sciences and disorders Contents: Communications science -- Communication disorders and the professions -- Anatomic processes of speech and hearing -- Child language disorders -- Child phonological disorders -- Fluency disorders -- Cleft lip and palate -- Voice disorders -- Neurogenic communication disorders -- Dysphagia -- Genetics and syndromes -- Hearing disorders -- Auditory rehabilitation. Subjects: Communicative disorders. Speech therapy. Audiology. Communication Disorders. Hearing Disorders. Notes: Includes bibliographical references and index.

Laryngeal diseases: symptoms, diagnosis and treatments LCCN: 2009031998 Main title: Laryngeal diseases: symptoms, diagnosis and treatments / Oldrich Nemecek and Viktor Mares, editors. Published/Created: Hauppauge, NY: Nova Science, c2010. Description: 171 p.: ill. (some col.); 26 cm. ISBN: 9781608761074 (hardcover: alk. paper) LC classification: RF510 .L357 2010 Related names: Nemecek, Oldrich, 1956- Mares, Viktor. Contents: Psychogenic voice disorders / Grace W. Johnson ... [et al.] -- Effects of vocal training on quantitative voice parameters in healthy voice adults and children / Nora Siupsinskiene -- Laryngeal squamous cell carcinoma: treatment options and outcomes / William M. Mendenhall ... [et al.] -- Endoscopic laser microsurgery of malignant tumors of the larynx: perioperative and postoperative complications / Maik Ellies -- Role of non-acidic reflux in laryngeal injury and disease /

Nikki Johnston -- Age as a factor in responses to botulinum toxin injection in adductor spasmodic dysphonia patients / Christopher Y. Chang ... [et al.] -- The importance of the autofluorescence and contact endoscopy in the diagnosis of laryngeal lesions / Marcin Fraczek, Maciej Zatonski, Tomasz Krecicki -- Electroglottography in follow-up of patients with vocal fold palsy / Olaf Zagólski -- Laryngeal problems in patients suffering from rheumatoid arthritis / Katarzyna Amernik ... [et al.] -- Alcohol-related comorbidity measurement in patients with laryngeal squamous cell carcinoma / Mario A.F. Castro ... [et al.]. Subjects: Larynx--Diseases. Laryngeal Diseases--therapy. Laryngeal Diseases--diagnosis. Notes: Includes bibliographical references and index. Series: Otolaryngology research advances.

Mosby's review questions for the speech-language pathology Praxis examination LCCN: 2009035660 Main title: Mosby's review questions for the speech-language pathology Praxis examination / edited by Dennis M. Ruscello. Published/Created: Maryland Heights, Mo.: Mosby/Elsevier, c2010. Description: xii, 363 p.; 28 cm. + 1 CD-ROM (4 3/4 in.) ISBN: 9780323059046 (pbk.: alk. paper) 032305904X (pbk.: alk. paper) LC classification: RC423 .M598 2010 Portion of title: Review questions for the speech-language pathology Praxis examination Related names: Ruscello, Dennis M. Contents: Language acquisition and cognition / Paula Menyuk -- Language science / Lisa Hammett Price and Yvette D. Hyter -- Learning theory / Steven L. Skelton -- Multicultural awareness / Kay T. Payne -- Speech science / Richard D. Andreatta -- Phonological disorders / Benjamin Munson -- Child language disorders / Patricia A. Prelock and Diana B. Newman -- Fluency disorders / Tommie L. Robinson -- Resonance disorders / David L. Jones -- Voice disorders / Joseph Stemple, Ashwini Joshi, and Anysia Ensslen -- Neurological disorders / Carl Coelho ... [et al.] -- Dysphagia / JoAnne Robbins ... [et al.] -- Hearing science / John A. Ferraro -- Audiological assessment / Ashleigh A. Payne -- Auditory habilitation and rehabilitation / Nancy Tye-Murray -- Alternative and augmentative communication / Kathleen Franklin -- Counseling

/ Audrey L. Holland -- Documentation and monitoring of patient progress / Leslie C. Graebe and Karen B. Haines -- Efficacy / Mary Pannbacker -- Instrumentation / J. Anthony Seikel -- Speech-language assessment / Karen B. Haines and Leslie C. Graebe -- Speech-language intervention / Betsy Partin Vinson -- Syndromes and genetics / Linda D. Vallino -- Ethical practices / David L. Irwin -- Research methodology and psychometrics / Susan Rvachew -- Standards and laws / Shelly S. Chabon and Dorian Lee-Wilkerson. Subjects: Speech therapy--Examinations, questions, etc. Speech-Language Pathology--Examination Questions. Notes: Includes bibliographical references and index.

Occupational emergency medicine LCCN: 2010027212 Main title: Occupational emergency medicine / edited by Michael I. Greenberg; associate editor, James M. Madsen. Published/Created: Oxford; Hoboken, NJ: Wiley-Blackwell, 2011. Description: vii, 280 p.: ill. (some col.); 25 cm. Links: Contributor biographical information http://catdir.loc.gov/catdir/enhancements/fy1013/2010027212-b.html Publisher description http://catdir.loc.gov/catdir/enhancements/fy1013/2010027212-d.html Table of contents only http://catdir.loc.gov/catdir/enhancements/fy1013/2010027212-t.html ISBN: 9781405180719 1405180714 LC classification: RC964 .O253 2011 Related names: Greenberg, Michael I. Madsen, James M. Contents: Potentially lethal occupational exposures / Christina Price and Dennis P. Price -- Occupational dermatology: issues for the emergency department / David Vearrier -- Occupational infections / Amy J. Behrman -- Occupational toxicology / John Curtis and David A. Haggerty -- Work-related trauma and injury / Mark Saks and Brad Rahaman -- Occupationally based disaster medicine / James M. Madsen -- Work-related ocular injuries / Joseph L. D'Orazio -- Occupational illness and injury in law enforcement personnel / Richard Tovar -- Occupational illness and injury in firefighters / Richard Tovar -- Occupational illness and injury in prehospital care personnel / Derek Isenberg and Carin Van Gelder -- Occupational pulmonary disease / Michael G. Holland -- Health hazards and emergency care for health care workers / Amy J. Behrman -- Occupational concerns for truckers and drivers / Natalie P. Hartenbaum -- Arts medicine: an overview for emergency physicians / Robert T. Sataloff and Mary J. Hawkshaw -- Occupational hearing loss: an overview for emergency physicians / Robert T. Sataloff, Mary J. Hawkshaw, and Joseph Sataloff -- Voice disorders: an overview for emergency physicians / Robert T. Sataloff and Mary J. Hawkshaw -- Unusual problems in occupational emergency medicine / Edward A. Ramoska and Guneesh Saluja. Subjects: Occupational diseases. Medical emergencies. Industrial toxicology. Toxicological emergencies. Emergencies. Occupational Diseases--therapy. Accidents, Occupational. Emergency Service, Hospital. Occupational Exposure--adverse effects. Notes: Includes bibliographical references and index.

Pediatric voice: a modern, collaborative approach to care LCCN: 2013035348 Personal name: Kelchner, Lisa N., author. Main title: Pediatric voice: a modern, collaborative approach to care / Lisa N. Kelchner, Susan Baker Brehm, Barbara Weinrich. Published/Produced: San Diego, CA: Plural Publishing, [2014] Description: p.; cm. ISBN: 9781597564625 (alk. paper) 1597564621 (alk. paper) LC classification: RF510 Related names: Brehm, Susan Baker, author. Weinrich, Barbara Derickson, author. Contents: Anatomy and physiology of the pediatric upper aerodigestive tract, larynx, and respiratory system -- Neural controls of voice -- Etiology and management of pediatric voice disorders (contributed by Alessandro de Alarcon) -- A collaborative approach to evaluating the child with a voice disorder -- A collaborative approach to treatment -- Managing children with complex voice disorders. Subjects: Voice Disorders--diagnosis. Child. Voice--physiology. Voice Disorders--therapy. Notes: Includes bibliographical references and index.

Professional voice: assessment and management: proceedings of the National Workshop on Professional Voice: Assessment and Management, 9-10 December, 2010 LCCN: 2010317587 Meeting name: National Workshop on Professional Voice: Assessment and Management (2010: All India Institute of Speech &

Hearing) Main title: Professional voice: assessment and management: proceedings of the National Workshop on Professional Voice: Assessment and Management, 9-10 December, 2010 / editor, Vijayalakshmi Basavaraj. Published/Created: Mysore: All India Institute of Speech & Hearing, 2010. Description: iii, 117 pages: illustrations; 25 cm LC classification: RF510 .N37 2010 Related names: Basavaraj, Vijayalakshmi, editor of compilation. All India Institute of Speech and Hearing, host institution. Subjects: Voice disorders--Prevention--Congresses. Voice--Care and hygiene--Congresses. Notes: Includes bibliographical references.

Singing voice rehabilitation: a guide for the voice teacher and speech-language pathologist LCCN: 2009935142 Personal name: Wicklund, Karen. Main title: Singing voice rehabilitation: a guide for the voice teacher and speech-language pathologist / Karen Wicklund. Published/Created: Clifton Park, NY: Delmar, c2010. Description: xxi, 241 p.: ill. (some col.), forms; 26 cm. Links: Contributor biographical information http://www.loc.gov/catdir/enhancements/fy1303/2009935142-b.html Publisher description http://www.loc.gov/catdir/enhancements/fy1303/2009935142-d.html Table of contents only http://www.loc.gov/catdir/enhancements/fy1303/2009935142-t.html ISBN: 9781435438545 143543854X LC classification: RF511.S55 W53 2010 Contents: Normal voice: anatomy and physiology -- Vocal injuries and their effect on vocal parameters -- Psychosocial effects of singing voice loss -- Vocal outcome tracks for singers -- Singer's voice care team: quality care through specialization and collaboration -- Creating an individualized singing voice therapy protocol -- Therapeutic song repertoire: classical and musical theater -- Special considerations for the vocally injured student singer -- Taking steps to preventing vocal reinjury -- Future of singing voice rehabilitation as a profession. Subjects: Voice disorders--Treatment. Voice--physiology. Voice Disorders--rehabilitation. Music. Occupational Diseases. Notes: Includes bibliographical references (p. 229-234) and index.

Speech and language challenges: the ultimate teen guide LCCN: 2014007973 Personal name: Brill, Marlene Targ. Main title: Speech and language challenges: the ultimate teen guide / Marlene Targ Brill. Published/Produced: Lanham: Rowman & Littlefield, [2014] ©2014 Description: xiii, 227 pages: illustrations; 26 cm. ISBN: 9780810887916 (cloth: alk. paper) 0810887916 (cloth: alk. paper) LC classification: RJ496.C67 B75 2014 Contents: The amazing story of communication -- When words won't flow: stuttering and other fluency challenges -- Mixed-up sounds and words: speech sound disorders -- When the voice goes haywire: voice disorders -- When the brain hears and processes infomation differntly: language disorders -- Cars, guns, sports, adn the unexpected: brain injury and communication -- When English is new or sounds different -- Technology as a communication game changer -- Looking ahead: boosting communications skills all around. Subjects: Communicative disorders in adolescence. Notes: Includes bibliographical references (pages 211-221) and index. Grades 9-12. Series: It happened to me; no. 40.

Speech disorders: causes, treatment and social effects LCCN: 2009031120 Main title: Speech disorders: causes, treatment and social effects / editor, Alan E. Harrison. Published/Created: Hauppauge, N.Y.: Nova Science Publishers, Inc., c2010. Description: xiv, 329 p.: ill.; 26 cm. ISBN: 9781608762132 (hardcover: alk. paper) LC classification: RC423 .S63827 2010 Related names: Harrison, Alan E. Contents: Preface -- Speech and voice disorders in Parkinson's Disease / Sabine Skodda -- Speech and Literacy: The Connection and the Relevance to Clinical Populations / Jonathan L. Preston -- Imaging of Brain Function with Positron Emission Tomography and its Role in Aphasia Research / Wolf-Dieter Heiss -- Using Spanish in the Home to Promote School Readiness in English / Virginia Mann, Maricela Sandoval, Lorena Garcia, David Calderon -- New Frontiers in Understanding Speech Sound Disorder: Unraveling the Mysteries of Genetic Causes / Beate Peter -- Treatment Outcomes of the Intensive Stuttering Therapy for Adolescents and Adults / Rodney Gabel, Farzan Irani, Scott Palasik, Eric Swartz,

Charlie Hughes -- Is Prosody a Diagnostic and Cognitive Bellwether of Autism Spectrum Disorders? / Joshua John Diehl, Lauren D. Berkovits -- The Multi Dimensional Voice Program (MDVP) in Conjunction with Other Tests in the Evaluation of Speech and Voice Disorders: Our Experience / A. Salami, R. Mora, B. Crippa, M. Dellepiane, B. Jankowska -- Learning Disabilities and Mathematics in Higher Education / Brian Watson, Stuart Rowlands -- Speech Evaluation and Speech Rehabilitation after Oral and Oropharyngeal Cancer Treatment / Viviane de Carvalho-Teles, Ingrid Gielow -- Audience Effects on Stuttering: A Japanese Case Study / Jun Yamada, Takanobu Homma -- Silent Children: Understanding and Treating Selective Mutism / Katharina Manassis -- Effectiveness of Speech Rate-Conversion Software for Patients with Dysarthria / Masaki Nishio, Yasuhiro Tanaka, Chikako Sakabibara, Naoko Abe -- Speech Problems in Dyslexia: Evidence from Auditory and Visual Speech Perception / Joshua Ramirez, Virginia Mann -- Index. Subjects: Speech disorders. Language disorders. Communicative disorders. Notes: Includes bibliographical references and index.

Speech, language and voice pathology: methods, challenges and outcomes LCCN: 2014034866 Main title: Speech, language and voice pathology: methods, challenges and outcomes / Pablo Antonio Ysunza, editor. Published/Produced: New York: Nova Publishers, [2014] ©2014 Description: ix, 184 pages: illustrations; 24 cm. ISBN: 9781633219588 (hardcover) 1633219585 (hardcover) LC classification: RC423 .S6394 2014 Related names: Ysunza, Pablo Antonio, editor of compilation. Subjects: Speech disorders. Language disorders. Voice disorders. Notes: Includes bibliographical references and index. Series: Languages and linguistics.

Stroboscopy LCCN: 2009024123 Personal name: Woo, Peak. Main title: Stroboscopy / Peak Woo. Published/Created: San Diego: Plural Pub., c2010. Description: xvi, 385 p.: ill. (some col.); 29 cm. ISBN: 9781597560146 (alk. paper) 1597560146 (alk. paper) LC classification: RF514.5 .W66 2010 Subjects:

Laryngostroboscopy. Voice disorders--Diagnosis. Laryngeal Diseases--diagnosis. Vocal Cords--physiopathology. Stroboscopy--methods. Vocal Cords--physiology. Notes: Includes bibliographical references and index.

The Cambridge handbook of communication disorders LCCN: 2013018451 Main title: The Cambridge handbook of communication disorders / edited by Louise Cummings. Published/Produced: Cambridge: Cambridge University Press, 2014. Description: xxiv, 690 pages: illustrations; 26 cm. Links: Cover image http://assets.cambridge.org/97811070/21235/cover/9781107021235.jpg ISBN: 9781107021235 (hardback) LC classification: RC423 .C24 2014 Related names: Cummings, Louise. Summary: "Many children and adults experience impairment of their communication skills. These communication disorders impact adversely on all aspects of these individuals' lives. In thirty dedicated chapters, The Cambridge Handbook of Communication Disorders examines the full range of developmental and acquired communication disorders and provides the most up-to-date and comprehensive guide to the epidemiology, aetiology and clinical features of these disorders. The volume also examines how these disorders are assessed and treated by speech and language therapists and addresses recent theoretical developments in the field. The handbook goes beyond well-known communication disorders to include populations such as children with emotional disturbance, adults with non-Alzheimer dementias and people with personality disorders. Each chapter describes in accessible terms the most recent thinking and research in communication disorders. The volume is an ideal guide for academic researchers, graduate students and professionals in speech and language therapy"-- Provided by publisher. Contents: Machine generated contents note: Part I. Developmental Communication Disorders: 1. Cleft lip and palate and other craniofacial anomalies -- John E. Riski; 2. Developmental dysarthria -- Megan Hodge; 3. Developmental verbal dyspraxia -- Brigid McNeill; 4. Developmental phonological disorder -- Susan Rvachew; 5. Specific language impairment -- Susan Ellis Weismer; 6. Developmental dyslexia --

Catherine Christo; 7. Intellectual disability and communication -- Katherine Short-Meyerson and Glenis Benson; 8. Emotional disturbance and communication -- Gregory J. Benner and J. Ron Nelson; 9. Autistic spectrum disorders and communication -- Courtenay Frazier Norbury; Part II. Acquired Communication Disorders: 10. Head and neck cancer and communication -- Tim Bressmann; 11. Acquired dysarthria -- Bruce E. Murdoch; 12. Apraxia of speech -- Donald A. Robin and Sabina Flagmeier; 13. Aphasia -- Roelien Bastiaanse and Ronald S. Prins; 14. Right hemisphere damage and communication -- Yves Joanette, Perrine Ferre; and Maximiliano A. Wilson; 15. Dementia and communication -- Jamie Reilly and Jinyi Hung; 16. Traumatic brain injury and communication -- Leanne Togher; 17. Psychiatric disorders and communication -- Karen Bryan; Part III. Voice, Fluency and Hearing Disorders: 18. Functional and organic voice disorders -- Nadine P. Connor and Diane M. Bless; 19. Stuttering and cluttering -- Kathleen Scaler Scott; 20. Hearing disorders -- R. Steven Ackley; Part IV. Management of Communication Disorders: 21. Developmental motor speech disorders -- Kirrie J. Ballard and Patricia McCabe; 22. Acquired motor speech disorders -- Anja Lowitt; 23. Developmental language disorders -- Laurence B. Leonard; 24. Acquired aphasia -- Anne Whitworth, Janet Webster and Julie Morris; 25. Disorders of voice -- Linda Rammage; 26. Disorders of fluency -- J. Scott Yaruss; Part V. Theoretical Developments in Communication Disorders: 27. Motor speech disorders and models of speech production -- Karen Croot; 28. Adult neurological disorders and semantic models -- Tobias Bormann; 29. Language in genetic syndromes and cognitive modularity -- Vesna Stojanovik; 30. Pragmatic disorders and theory of mind -- Louise Cummings. Subjects: Communicative disorders--Handbooks, manuals, etc. LANGUAGE ARTS & DISCIPLINES / Linguistics / General. Notes: Includes bibliographical references and index. Series: Cambridge handbooks in language and linguistics.

The communication disorders workbook LCCN: 2013037707 Personal name: Cummings, Louise, author. Main title: The communication disorders workbook / Louise Cummings. Published/Produced: Cambridge; New York: Cambridge University Press, 2014. Description: xiv, 211 pages 26 cm. ISBN: 9781107054981 (hardback) 1107054982 (hardback) 9781107633414 (pbk.) 1107633419 (pbk.) LC classification: RC428 .C86 2014 Contents: Introduction to communication disorders -- Developmental speech disorders -- Developmental language disorders -- Communication disorders in mental illness -- Acquired speech disorders -- Acquired language disorders -- Disorders of voice -- Disorders of fluency -- Hearing disorders. Subjects: Language Disorders--Case Reports. Language Disorders--Programmed Instruction. Communication Disorders--Case Reports. Communication Disorders--Programmed Instruction. Notes: Includes bibliographical references and index.

The handbook of language and speech disorders LCCN: 2009030171 Main title: The handbook of language and speech disorders / edited by Jack S. Damico, Nicole Müller, and Martin J. Ball. Published/Created: Malden, Mass.: Wiley-Blackwell, 2010. Description: p. cm. ISBN: 9781405158626 (hardcover: alk. paper) 9781118347164 (pbk.) LC classification: RC423 .H3258 2010 Related names: Damico, Jack, 1952- Müller, Nicole, 1963- Ball, Martin J. (Martin John) Contents: List of figures -- Notes on contributors -- Introduction / Jack S. Damico, Nicole Müller and Martin J. Ball -- Part I. Foundations: 1. Social and Practial Considerations in Labeling / Jack S. Damico, Nicole Müller, and Martin J. Ball -- 2. Diversity Considerations in Speech and Language Disorders / Brian A. Goldstein and Ramonda Horton-Ikard -- 3. Intervention for Children with Auditory or Visual Sensory Impairments / Laura W. Kretschmer and Richard. R. Kretschmer -- 4. Intelligibility Impairments / Megan Hodge and Tara Whitehill -- 5. Genetic Syndromes and Communication Disorders / Vesna Stojanovik -- 6. Principles of Assessment and Intervention / Bonnie Brinton and Martin Fujiki -- Part II. Language Disorders: 7. Autism Spectrum Disorders: The State of the Art / John Muma and Steven Cloud -- 8. Delayed Language Development in Preschool Children / Deborah Weiss and Rhea Paul -- 9.

Specific Language Impairment / Sandra L. Gillam and Alan G. Kamhi -- 10. Pragmatic Impairment / Michael R. Perkins -- 11. Learning Disabilities / Robert Reid and Laura Jacobson -- 12. Reading and Reading Impairments / Jack S. Damico and Ryan Nelson -- 13. Substance Abuse and Childhood Language Disorders / Truman E. Coggins and John C. Thorne -- 14. Aphasia / Chris F. S. Code -- Part III. Speech Disorders: 15. Children with Speech Sound Disorders / Sara Howard -- 16. Dysarthria / Hermann Ackermann, Ingo Hertrich, and Wolfram Ziegler -- 17. Apraxia of Speech / Adam Jacks and Donald A. Robin -- 18. Augmentative and Alternative Communication: An Introduction / Kathryn D. R. Drager, Erinn F. Finke, and Elizabeth C. Serpentine -- 19. Fluency and Fluency Disorders / John A. TeTnowski and Kathy Scaler Scott -- 20. describing voice disorders / Richard Morris and Archie Bernard Harmon -- 21. Orofacial Anomalies / Jane Russell -- 22. Speech Disorders Related to Head and Neck Cancer: Laryngectomy, Glossectomy, and Velopharyngeal and Maxillofacial Defects / Tim Bressmann -- Part IV. Cognitive and Intellectual Disorders: 23. ADHD and Communication Disorders / Carol Westby and Silvana Watson -- 24. Communication Deficits Associated with Right Hemisphere Brain Damage / Margaret Lehman Blake -- 25. Traumatic Brain Injury / Jennifer Mozeiko, Karen Lé and Carl Coelho -- 26. Dementia / Nicole Müller -- Author Index -- Subject Index. Subjects: Speech disorders. Language disorders. Communicative disorders. Notes: Includes bibliographical references and index. Series: Blackwell handbooks in linguistics.

The manual of speech sound disorders: a book for students and clinicians LCCN: 2013953466 Personal name: Bleile, Ken Mitchell, author. Uniform title: Manual of articulation and phonological disorders Main title: The manual of speech sound disorders: a book for students and clinicians / Ken M. Bleile. Edition: Third edition. Published/Produced: Stamford, CT: Cengage Learning, [2015] ©2015 Description: xii, 451 pages; 24 cm + 1 CD-ROM (4 3/4 in.) Links: Contributor biographical information http://www.loc.gov/catdir/enhan

cements/fy1503/2013953466-b.html Publisher description http://www.loc.gov/catdir/enhancements/fy1503/2013953466-d.html Table of contents only http://www.loc.gov/catdir/enhancements/fy1503/2013953466-t.html ISBN: 9781111313784 1111313784 9781285175539 1285175530 LC classification: RC424.7 .B56 2014 Portion of title: Speech sound disorders Contents: Machine generated contents note: 1. FOUNDATIONS -- ch. 1 Speech and Its Disorders -- ch. 2 Terminology -- ch. 3 Speech Variations -- 2. SPEECH DEVELOPMENT -- ch. 4 The Neurology of Speech Learning -- ch. 5 Infants -- ch. 6 Toddlers -- ch. 7 Preschoolers -- ch. 8 School-Age Students -- ch. 9 Summary of Speech Development -- 3. ASSESSMENT -- ch. 10 Assessment of Communication -- ch. 11 Hypothesis Testing -- ch. 12 Data Collection -- ch. 13 Analysis -- ch. 14 Published Tests -- 4. TREATMENT -- ch. 15 Treatment Principles -- ch. 16 Goals -- ch. 17 Treatment Sounds -- ch. 18 Talking with Children -- ch. 19 Talking About Speech -- ch. 20 Phonetic Placement and Shaping -- ch. 21 Treatment Approaches -- ch. 22 Treatment Activities. Subjects: Articulation disorders. Voice disorders. Articulation Disorders--diagnosis--Handbook. Articulation disorders. Form/Genre: Handbooks, manuals, etc. Notes: Revision of: Manual of articulation and phonological disorders: infancy through adulthood. Includes bibliographical references and index.

The voice and voice therapy LCCN: 2008043476 Personal name: Boone, Daniel R. Main title: The voice and voice therapy / Daniel R. Boone ... [et al.]. Edition: 8th ed. Published/Created: Boston: Allyn and Bacon, c2010. Description: xvi, 344 p.: ill.; 23 cm. + 1 videodisc (DVD: sd., col.; 4 3/4 in.) ISBN: 9780205609536 (hardcover) 0205609538 (hardcover) LC classification: RF540 .B66 2010 Subjects: Voice disorders--Textbooks. Notes: Includes bibliographical references (p. 307-334) and index.

The voice and voice therapy LCCN: 2012050999 Personal name: Boone, Daniel R. Main title: The voice and voice therapy / Daniel R. Boone, University of Arizona, Stephen C. McFarlane, University of Nevada Medical School, Shelley L. von Berg,

California State University, Chico, Richard I. Zraick, University of Arkansas for Medical Sciences/University of Arkansas at Little Rock. Edition: Ninth edition. Published/Produced: Boston: Pearson, [2014] Description: xix, 636 pages: illustrations some color; 27 cm ISBN: 9780133007022 0133007022 LC classification: RF540 .B66 2014 Related names: McFarlane, Stephen C. Von Berg, Shelley L. Zraick, Richard I., 1962- Subjects: Voice disorders--Textbooks. Notes: Includes bibliographical references (pages 321-356) and index.

Understanding voice problems: a physiological perspective for diagnosis and treatment LCCN: 2010045739 Personal name: Colton, Raymond H., author. Main title: Understanding voice problems: a physiological perspective for diagnosis and treatment / Raymond H. Colton, Janina K. Casper, Rebecca Leonard. Edition: Fourth edition. Published/Created: Philadelphia: Wolters Kluwer Health/Lippincott Williams & Wilkins, [2011], ©2011. Description: xi, 494 pages: illustrations; 26 cm Links: Publisher description http://www.loc.gov/catdir/enhancements/fy1201/2010045739-d.html Table of contents only http://www.loc.gov/catdir/enhancements/fy1201/2010045739-t.html ISBN: 9781609138745 (hardback: alkaline paper) 1609138740 LC classification: RF510 .C65 2011 Related names: Casper, Janina K., author. Leonard, Rebecca, author. Summary: "Understanding Voice Problems: A Physiological Perspective for Diagnosis and Treatment emphasizes the physiological perspective of voice disorders and the behavioral and emotional factors that can influence these changes. Readers will find a strong foundation in normal phonatory physiology and acoustics as well as pathophysiology arising from voice misuse, abuse, or neurological involvement. Coverage includes in-depth explorations of patient interviewing, history-taking, examination, and testing and discussions of pediatric and geriatric voice considerations. The book contains numerous illustrations, including full-color plates of vocal fold pathologies. A companion Website features nearly 30 video clips that demonstrate healthy, normally functioning larynges at work, plus larynges with various pathological problems"-- Provided by publisher. Contents: Machine generated contents note: Color plates precede page i Preface 1 Introduction and Overview 2 Differential Diagnosis of Voice Problems 3 Morphology of Vocal Fold Mucosa: Histology to Genomics 4 Phonotrauma: Its Effects on Phonatory Physiology 5 Voice Problems Associated With Nervous System Involvement 6 Voice Problems Associated With Organic Disease and Trauma 7 Voice Problems Associated With the Pediatric and the Geriatric Voice 8 The Voice History, Examination, and Testing 9 Surgical and Medical Management of Voice Disorders 10 Vocal Rehabilitation 11 Anatomy of the Vocal Fold Mechanism 12 Phonatory Physiology 13 Neuroanatomy of the Vocal Mechanism 14 Some Normative Data on the Voice Appendix: Forms Used in Voice Evaluation: Clinic and Laboratory References Figure and Table Credits Index . Subjects: Voice disorders--Pathophysiology. Voice Disorders--physiopathology. Voice Disorders--therapy. Larynx--physiology. Voice Disorders--diagnosis. Notes: Includes bibliographical references (pages 435-469) and index.

Voice and communication therapy for the transgender/transsexual client: a comprehensive clinical guide LCCN: 2012000440 Main title: Voice and communication therapy for the transgender/transsexual client: a comprehensive clinical guide / edited by Richard K. Adler, Sandy Hirsch, Michelle Mordaunt. Edition: 2nd ed. Published/Created: San Diego, CA: Plural Pub., c2012. Description: xxi, 551 p.: ill.; 23 cm + 1 sound disc (digital; 4 3/4 in.) ISBN: 9781597564700 (alk. paper) 1597564702 (alk. paper) LC classification: RF511.T73 V65 2012 Related names: Adler, Richard Kenneth. Hirsch, Sandy. Mordaunt, Michelle. Contents: A historical perspective and review of the literature / Jack Pickering and Lauren Baker -- A team approach: the role of the clinician / Celia R. Hooper and Laura Tallant -- Evidence-based practice / Jennifer Oates -- Psychosocial issues / Richard K. Adler and Alice Christianson -- Psychotherapy: revisited / Randi Ettner -- Assessment and goal setting: revisited / Georgia Dacakis -- Vocal health and phonotrauma / Richard K. Adler and Christella Antoni -- Female to male considerations / Richard Adler, Alex N. Constansis, and John Van Borsel -- Pitch and intonation / Marylou P. Gelfer and Michelle Mordaunt -- Resonance / Sandy Hirsch and Marylou P. Gelfer -- Articulation / Joan Boonin -- Rate and volume / Joan Boonin -- Language: pragmatics and discourse / Ashley M. Frazier and Celia R. Hooper -- Language: syntax and semantics: a menu of communicative choices / Celia R. Hooper, Sena Crutchley and Vicki McCready -- Nonverbal communication: multicultural issues / Sandy Hirsch and John Van Borsel -- Nonverbal communication: assessment and training / Sandy Hirsch and Joan Boonin -- Group therapy / Michelle Mordaunt -- The singing voice / Anita Kozan -- Theatrical meanderings: an interview: Sandy Hirsch with Rebecca M. Root / Sandy Hirsch and Rebecca M. Root -- Considerations for discharge and maintenance / Michelle Mordaunt and Sandy Hirsch -- Summary / Michelle Mordaunt. Subjects: Voice disorders--Treatment. Communicative disorders--Treatment. Sex change--Complications. Transgender people--Health and hygiene. Transsexuals--Health and hygiene. Transgender people--Mental health. Transsexuals--Mental health. Voice Training. Nonverbal Communication. Transsexualism. Voice Quality. Notes: Includes bibliographical references and index.

Voice disorders LCCN: 2012032271 Personal name: Sapienza, Christine M. Main title: Voice disorders / Christine Sapienza and Bari Hoffman Ruddy. Edition: 2nd ed. Published/Created: San Diego: Plural Pub., c2013. Description: xv, 379 p.: ill. (some col.); 26 cm + 1 DVD (4 3/4 in.) ISBN: 9781597564939 (pbk.: alk. paper) 1597564931 (pbk.: alk. paper) LC classification: RF510 .S25 2013 Related names: Hoffman Ruddy, Bari. Subjects: Voice Disorders. Notes: Includes bibliographical references and index.

Voice disorders: scope of theory and practice LCCN: 2011021054 Personal name: Ferrand, Carole T. Main title: Voice disorders: scope of theory and practice / Carole T. Ferrand. Published/Created: Boston: Pearson, c2012. Description: xxiii, 551 p.: ill. (some col.); 26 cm. ISBN: 9780205540532 (casebound) 0205540538 (casebound) LC classification: RF510 .F49 2012 Contents: Anatomy and physiology of the respiratory and laryngeal systems -- Lifespan changes in the respiratory and phonatory systems -- Considerations in voice treatment -- Diagnosis and evaluation of voice disorders -- Clinical management -- Inflammatory conditions of the larynx -- Structural lesions of the larynx -- Benign lesions of the vocal fold mucosa and vocal fatigue associated with lifestyle, personality, and occupational factors -- Movement disorders -- Voice disorders related to self and identity -- Disorders related to airway problems and respiration -- Laryngeal cancer. Subjects: Voice disorders. Voice Disorders. Respiration. Respiratory Tract Diseases. Notes: Includes bibliographical references and indexes. Series: The Allyn & Bacon communication sciences and disorders series Allyn & Bacon communication sciences and disorders series.

Voice therapy: clinical case studies LCCN: 2009036442 Main title: Voice therapy: clinical case studies / [edited by] Joseph C. Stemple and Lisa Fry. Edition: 3rd ed. Published/Created: San Diego: Plural Pub., c2010. Description: xix, 453 p.: ill.; 26 cm. ISBN: 9781597563444 (alk. paper) 1597563447 (alk. paper) LC classification: RF510 .V68 2010 Related names: Stemple, Joseph C. Thomas Fry, Lisa. Contents: Principles of voice therapy / Joseph C. Stemple -- Comments on the voice evaluation / Joseph C. Stemple -- Management of vocal hyperfunction and associated pathologies -- Management of glottal incompetence -- Management of functional voice disorders -- Irritable larynx syndrome and respiratory disorders -- Management of the professional voice -- Management approaches for neurogenic voice disorders -- Successful voice therapy / Joseph C. Stemple and Eva van Lear. Subjects: Voice disorders--Treatment. Voice Disorders--therapy--Case Reports. Notes: Includes bibliographical references and index.

Voice therapy: clinical case studies LCCN: 2014000154 Main title: Voice therapy: clinical case studies / [edited by] Joseph C. Stemple, PhD, CCC-SLP, ASHAF, Edie R. Hapner, PhD, CCC-SLP. Edition: Fourth edition. Published/Produced: San Diego, CA: Plural Publishing, Inc., [2014] ©2014

Description: xxiv, 530 pages: illustrations; 26 cm ISBN: 9781597565585 (alk. paper) 159756558X (alk. paper) LC classification: RF510 .V68 2014 Related names: Stemple, Joseph C., editor of compilation. Hapner, Edie R., editor of compilation. Contents: Principles of voice therapy / Joseph C. Stemple -- Comments on the voice evaluation / Joseph C. Stemple -- Primary and secondary muscle tension dysphonia -- Management of glottal incompetence -- Dystonia, essential tremor, and other neurogenic disorders -- Irritable larynx syndrome, paradoxical vocal fold dysfunction, and chronic cough -- Management of the professional, avocational, and occupational voice -- Successful voice therapy. Subjects: Voice disorders--Treatment. Voice Disorders--therapy--Case Reports. Notes: Includes bibliographical references and index.

Your voice at its best: enhancement of the healthy voice for the troubled voice LCCN: 2011456163 Personal name: McClosky, David Blair. Main title: Your voice at its best: enhancement of the healthy voice for the troubled voice / David Blair McClosky with members of the McClosky Institute of Voice. Edition: 5th ed. Published/Created: Long Grove, Ill.: Waveland Press Inc., c2011. Description: xii, 104 p.: ill. 23 cm. ISBN: 9781577667056 (pbk.) 1577667050 (pbk.) LC classification: QP306 .M18 2011 Related names: McClosky Institute of Voice. Contents: The McClosky technique: posture and breathing -- Freeing the voice through the McClosky "six areas of relaxation" -- Phonation -- Freeing the voice from song to speech -- Articulation of consonants in detail -- Vocalizing with the McClosky technique -- Resonance and color -- Expressiveness and the McClosky technique -- Care of the voice -- Voice disorders. Subjects: Voice. Notes: Includes bibliographical references.

INDEX

A

B

C

D

E

F

G

H

I

J

L

S

T

U

V

W